Praise for Jenn Trepeck and her podcast, *Salad With a Side of Fries*

You can tell that she's smarter than the average health expert. Trepeck confounds other health coaches who like to hook clients for a lifetime. My favorite attribute of Trepeck's is her focus on motivating listeners, not lecturing to them. She is not one of those wellness podcast hosts where "failure is not an option." Instead, she recognizes and conveys that making lifestyle, fitness, and diet changes is exceedingly hard. Look for small wins, she urges, and do not make perfectionism the enemy of gradual progress.

–Frank Racioppi, author and journalist

Life before was black and white; it was exhausting! I no longer feel guilty. The mindset shift has been dramatic. This is a much healthier approach.

–Amy B.

This is a whole new mindset; complete 180º for me. I'm listening to my body.

–Yana W.

I can't get enough of this podcast! Thank you, Jenn, for cracking me up and encouraging me to order fries with my salads! I love recommending your podcast to patients; you get them to take notice of their habits! Thank you; great stuff here!

–jkwkrause (via Apple Podcasts)

Is [insert food/exercise/habit here] healthy? Check out the *Salad With A Side of Fries* podcast. Jenn shares a knowledgeable, approachable, and entertaining guide to living a balanced and healthy life. Good Stuff.

–Joanne, MSH; executive chef and culinary nutritionist (via Apple Podcasts)

Jenn brings a super healthy approach to tackling the many food dilemmas and issues we all deal with daily. Her energy and knowledge on the subject matter are infectious, helping you make smarter choices and providing a laugh along the way. *Salad with a Side of Fries* is a refreshing spin on debunking all those food myths and wacky health tricks, while teaching us to not be so hard on ourselves!

–ajlb5 (via Apple Podcasts)

Jenn puts out great info, and she backs it with evidence while keeping it light-hearted and fun. I've always thought food should be enjoyed and can be healthy too! They don't have to be mutually exclusive, and Jenn shares this each and every week! Thanks again for the info, insight, practical steps, and fun!

–hemingwayhelfdozen (via Apple Podcasts)

Jenn Trepeck is the authority on health and nutrition! Every episode is jam-packed with valuable information to level up your nutrition and help you feel better. Plus, the podcast is just fun to listen to!

–AnnaDKornick (via Apple Podcasts)

Uncomplicating
Wellness

DITCH THE RULES.
QUIET THE NOISE.
RECLAIM YOUR LIFE.

JENN TREPECK

Library of Congress Control Number: 2025919179

ISBN: 978-1-969267-02-4 (paperback)
ISBN: 978-1-969267-03-1 (ebook)

Published by Twin Flames Studios

DISCLAIMER

This book is for educational purposes only and does not provide medical, psychological, or professional advice. The authors and publisher disclaim any liability for errors, omissions, or outcomes related to the use of the information contained herein. Views expressed are solely those of the individuals involved and do not represent any agency or organization.

For everyone who has ever asked me a question about nutrition, habits, fad diets, willpower, motivation, or supplements, and every wellness warrior ready to reclaim their health and wellbeing. Let's lock arms. You are worth it, and you deserve it. ~Happy Healthy!

Contents

PART III: Read the Signs

PART IV: But What About...

Author's Note

Before we dive in, a quick but important note: I am not a medical doctor, and this book is not intended to diagnose, treat, cure, or prevent any disease. If you have specific health concerns, please consult with a licensed healthcare provider you trust. There is a time and a place for professional medical care, probably more often than you think, and also less often than some would have you believe. The goal here is not to replace your doctor but to help you approach wellness with more clarity, confidence, and discernment. There's room for both.

This book reflects the same approach I take on my podcast, *Salad with a Side of Fries*: it's a distillation of research, years of coaching, and hard-earned wisdom presented in a way that's actionable, relatable, and (most importantly) not overwhelming. To keep things uncomplicated, I've chosen not to include foot-notes or lengthy academic citations. This isn't a textbook. Instead, I've pulled from credible research and my real-world experience to give you the most relevant insights without turning this into a homework assignment.

Think of this as "wellness without the weirdness"—science, strategy, and sanity delivered with compassion and candor. I hope this book helps you cut through the noise, build trust in yourself, and start making choices that work for you.

With that, let's get started.

–Jenn

Introduction
WTF is Wellness Anyway?

Why You Feel Like You're Doing Everything and Still Getting Nowhere

Wellness is everywhere.

It's in your inbox, your Instagram feed, your grocery cart. It's in the text your friend just sent you about the supplement she swears by and the podcast your coworker wants you to listen to on your next walk. It's the reason you bought that $14 smoothie that tasted vaguely like lawn.

You're not short on advice. You're drowning in it.

And somehow, after all of it—after the books and the programs and the protein powders—you're still not sure what being well actually means. You've tried being good. You've tracked. You've fasted. You've juiced. You've ordered the salad when you really wanted the fries. And some days, you just said screw it and got the fries anyway, then felt bad about it.

Meanwhile, the world around you is throwing contradictions like dodgeballs. Coffee is a superfood—no, it's inflammatory. Fat is bad—wait, actually fat is good, but only the right fats, and only on Tuesdays if you've worked out and fasted while standing on your head. You should meditate, hydrate, exfoliate, activate your glutes, and eliminate sugar but not fruit but maybe also fruit?

Yeah. It's exhausting. And confusing. And kind of infuriating. And here's the truth no one has ever told you (or you refuse to believe):

YOU are NOT the problem. The system is.

The wellness world has become a branding exercise. A performance. A billion-dollar industry where the loudest voices often know the least and the people with the most lived experience are told to just *try harder*.

Let's pause here, because if you're reading this, I know something about you already: You care. You're doing a lot. You're smart enough to spot the BS, and tired enough to wonder if any of it is worth it.

You've likely asked yourself, *Why does it feel like I'm doing everything and still getting nowhere?* That's the question this book was born from.

So if you've ever felt like wellness is a job you didn't apply for, a test you're failing, or a finish line that keeps moving—you're in the right place. Hi, friend.

Full disclosure: This book isn't a plan. It's a perspective shift. We're going to uncomplicate wellness. Let's start by asking a better question than, "Am I doing it right?" Let's ask, "What the hell is wellness anyway?"

What We've Been Sold

For most of us, wellness was never clearly defined.

It just kind of oozed into our lives. One doctor's visit here, one clickbait headline there. Maybe a Weight Watchers meeting in the '90s. A coworker who swears by celery juice. Your mom's voice reminding you not to eat after 7:00 p.m. The apps. The trackers. The rules you didn't make but somehow follow anyway.

And if we had to guess what wellness actually meant? Most people would say, "Be thin. Don't get sick. Follow the plan."

The truth is that a lot of the institutions and systems that shaped our understanding of health weren't trying to create wellness in the first place. They were trying to cut costs, sell products, and avoid liability. Or just make things easier for overworked doctors and teachers in overburdened systems.

Let's take a look at how this plays out:

Doctors (as we know them in the US with our Western healthcare system) are trained to treat symptoms and diseases, not build health. They're not taught how to help you feel your best; they're taught how to get you back to "not sick." And that's not their fault. It's the system they were trained in. One that rewards efficiency over exploration, treatment over prevention, and checklists over curiosity.

Insurance companies don't insure health; they insure disease management and the sustainability of the insurance company. What they'll cover isn't necessarily what's best for your body. It's what's billable through a diagnosis code. Their job is to mitigate financial risk, not to help you thrive. They're not your wellness partner, they're your safety net when things go off the rails. And even then, only sometimes.

The diet industry doesn't want you well; it wants you hooked. It thrives on your dissatisfaction. It's built on shame, sustained by yo-yo results, and padded by marketing that convinces you your body is a problem to be solved. It sells you a finish line, knowing full well it's a loop. And when the plan doesn't work long-term? It blames you, not the product or the plan.

Media and marketing aestheticize health and moralize thinness, selling you an airbrushed version of wellness that has more to do with filters than facts.

Government guidelines are shaped more by lobbyists, subsidies, and political compromises than science. Powerful people, companies, and dollars determine what's defined as "healthy," often at the cost of what's truly effective.

Tech and biohacking culture promise optimization but often create anxiety. When your body becomes a data set to fix, you lose sight of what it means to feel energized and confident, not just measure well.

So no, the systems aren't optimized for wellness. They're optimized for maintenance, compliance, and mass-scale simplicity. (And often, to put dollars in someone's pocket).

But you're not a mass-scale product. You're a person. With a body. With needs. With a life. And that's why so many of us—despite doing everything "right"—still feel off. Still feel tired. Still feel like health is something other people get to have.

Because we've been measuring what they told us. We've been chasing the outcomes they implied. And we've been using broken tools to try to fix ourselves.

But the problem was never you.

So, What Is Wellness?

Wellness is not a number. It's not a cleanse. It's not a moral ranking of who had the kale salad and who had the fries. It's not the absence of illness. It's not your insurance company's approval. And it's not your BMI.

Wellness is the energy to live your life. It's the ability to chase your kid up the hill and roll down it laughing. It's sleeping through the night without pain. It's walking into your closet and not dreading getting dressed. It's thinking about something other than food all day. It's having the bandwidth to show up—for your job, your family, your joy.

Wellness is being able to choose. Because when you don't feel well, you don't have options. You have obligations. You're reacting, surviving, running on fumes. Real wellness gives you freedom—mental, emotional, physical.

And guess what? *You* get to define what that looks like for you. That's the first radical shift: *Wellness* isn't a standard to meet; it's a relationship to build. And it has layers. Yes, there's the physical stuff: nutrition, sleep, movement, blood sugar, hormones, energy. There's also the mental and emotional stuff: stress, joy, purpose, connection. And the relational stuff: how you show up with people you love. And the practical stuff: time, money, support, survival.

It all counts. And it's all connected.

We've been taught to treat health like it lives in its own little circle. But real wellness? It's the circle around all the other circles. It's what allows you to show up in your life, not what takes you away from it.

This isn't about *balance*, which, let's be honest, is kind of a trap. It's about presence. It's about being where you are. Owning your choices. Building capacity, without guilt or shame.

That's why wellness can't be about rules. It has to be about discernment.

Not, *Am I doing it right?*

But, *Is this working for me?*

That's the filter we're building in this book. One that quiets the noise and helps you tune into your own signals. Because no physician, no influencer, no app, no algorithm knows your body better than you do. And once you start to learn its language? Everything changes.

The Personal Shift

If you've ever felt like you were just meant to struggle with food forever, I get it. I spent years on the carousel of dieting. On again, off again. Up five pounds, down ten. Trying the thing (*every* thing), following the rules, doing everything "right"—only to watch it stop working, again. And then it was on to the next plan. The next fix. The next list of foods I was "allowed" to eat.

It wasn't a journey. It was a saga. Dramatic. Exhausting. All-consuming. And the worst part? I thought it was normal. That this was just what life would be: counting, restricting, rebounding, obsessing.

Until it wasn't.

Everything started to change when I stopped focusing on the number on the scale and started asking a different question, *What is my body doing with the food I'm giving it?*

Not what's "good or bad." Not what's "clean or dirty." Not whether I "should" eat it. Just, *How does my body process this? What's happening underneath the surface?*

That one shift opened the door to the science behind the hype. To the biochemistry and the physiology. And more importantly, it gave me context. Suddenly, my cravings weren't moral failures; they were biological signals.

My "lack of discipline" wasn't a character flaw; it was a blood sugar crash. The plan didn't fail because I wasn't strong enough. The plan failed because it was never designed for real life—or real bodies—in the first place.

So I built a relationship with my body instead of trying to outsmart it. I stopped obsessing over food, not because I had stronger willpower, but because I finally understood what my body needed and why. And I reclaimed all the mental energy I had been spending on the "shoulds" and redirected it to the stuff that actually matters.

And now, as a coach and podcaster, that's the shift I help other people make too. Not toward perfection, but toward understanding, discernment, choice, and most importantly, toward real, sustainable wellness in every facet. Because when you stop trying to fix yourself and start learning to listen, you realize you were never broken.

This Book Is Your Filter

Let me be clear about something upfront: This is not a 30-day plan (or a 60- or 90-day plan). There are no gold stars. No weigh-ins. No before and after photos.

This isn't about following steps. It's about changing how you think, so you can stop following and start choosing for yourself.

Because once you can filter wellness advice through a smarter lens, you no longer need a new plan every Monday. You no longer need to feel guilty for skipping a workout or eating something you genuinely enjoy (even if it was someone else's birthday). You stop asking, *Is this allowed?* and start asking, *Is this working for me?*

This book is here to build that lens. It's a collection of principles, not prescriptions.

Each chapter unpacks a core truth that can help you untangle years of diet culture, shame marketing, hyped hacks, and one-size-fits-none advice. You don't have to read in order; just start where you are. Come back to what you need. Let each section be a conversation, not a command.

Some chapters will bust myths you didn't even know you were carrying. Others will zoom in on the things that actually move the needle. All of them will offer a mix of real talk and science delivered with humor, humanity, and just enough sass to keep it fun.

This isn't about doing wellness perfectly (now that we know what it is). It's about doing the pieces that work for you consistently enough to feel better (and better). It is about coming back to yourself so you can stop feeling like your health is a never-ending to-do list because wellness isn't a job.

It's your fuel. It's your foundation. It's your right. And you don't need anyone else's permission to reclaim it.

The Invitation

So let's bring it back to you. If you could change one thing about your health today or prevent one thing in the future, what would it be? Not ten things. Not everything. One. Write it down.

Now ask yourself, *What's standing in the way of doing it?* That's the task. Not to fix your whole life overnight. Not to nail the perfect routine. Just get honest about the gap. See it. That's where change starts, not with guilt, but with awareness.

And from here forward, that's how we'll move. Not with pressure, but with presence and trust in your body. Not with shoulds, but with practical strategies backed by science and common sense. Not with fear, but with curiosity and discernment.

Because wellness isn't about finally getting it "right." It's about finally making it yours. So let's quiet the noise, clear the fog, ditch the dogma, and uncomplicate your wellness.

You ready? Let's do this.

PART I

Quiet the Noise

1

You're the Magic Bullet

et's get one thing straight from the jump:

If you've ever wished for a magic bullet—some secret plan, miracle supplement, or perfect set of habits to finally "fix it"—this is going to be annoying and freeing all at once.

Because the magic bullet? It's you.

Yep. Not the diet. Not the app. Not the friend's cousin's shake program. You.

Now, before your brain chimes in with, "Cool, but then why haven't I figured it out yet?"—let's zoom out. You're not the problem. You've just spent years navigating a wellness world that sells solutions while quietly undermining your trust in yourself.

It's not a coincidence that you feel stuck. The system thrives when you do. Confused people are compliant people, and the wellness industry is good at keeping you confused. It speaks in urgent headlines and contradictory advice. Eat more protein, but not too much. Fast, but not for too long. Cut sugar, but enjoy life. Be consistent, but also flexible. Oh, and by the way? Start over on Monday.

It's no wonder you're exhausted. But here's the shift this chapter is inviting you into: the most powerful, sustainable, life-giving change won't come from finding a better system. It comes from learning to trust yourself inside this noisy one.

That's not a fluffy affirmation. It's a strategy. Because once you understand how this industry works—and how you've been conditioned to doubt yourself—you can stop waiting for the next fix and start filtering the nonsense. You can stop thinking you need someone else's plan and start remembering your own power.

This isn't about finally getting it "right." It's about reclaiming the ability to tell what's right for you.

The Problem Isn't You, It's the System

If you've ever felt like you "can't stick with anything," or like every attempt at getting healthier turns into a new version of the same old cycle—start strong, slip, shame, repeat—it's not because you lack willpower. It's because the wellness industry is structured to profit from your doubt.

Case in point: In 2019, the U.S. diet industry hit a record $78 billion. That's a lot of zeroes tied to people not reaching their goals. If diets worked, that industry wouldn't be booming. There would be a mass graduation ceremony of people who "figured it out" and left the game. But that's not what happens. Because what they're selling isn't solutions—it's control. And shame. And a cycle that keeps you trying the next thing instead of trusting yourself.

Meanwhile, what's happening to our actual health?

- Over 50 percent of US adults have diabetes
- 95 percent aren't getting enough fiber
- Only 12 percent of people are considered metabolically healthy
- And one in four dieters develops an eating disorder

Let's connect the dots. We're more informed than ever. Exercise is up. Smoking is down. People know what a macro is. And still, waistlines are growing, blood sugar is rising, and wellness feels harder than it needs to. That's not a personal failure. That's a system-level disconnect.

Because what you've been taught to chase—thinness, control, perfection—isn't health. And what you've been told to ignore, your hunger cues, your body's signals, your emotional wellbeing, is often the very thing you need to reclaim.

The result? You've spent years learning not to trust yourself. And in that space of doubt, the industry has filled the gap with rules, rigidity, and expensive "fixes."

Why the Fixes Keep Failing

Every diet, app, pill, or challenge you've tried had one thing in common: It told you the answer was out there. Something to follow. Something to obey. Something that would work if only you could keep up.

And when it didn't? It was quietly your fault.

Here's the truth: Those "fixes" weren't designed to create lasting change. They were designed to be compelling. To make you feel hopeful enough to start, and guilty enough to start over.

Let's break down a few of the greatest hits because naming them for what they are is step one in reclaiming your power.

Keto: All or Nothing with No Exit Strategy

Created initially as a clinical tool for pediatric epilepsy, keto wasn't built for your brunch plans or your biology. To maintain ketosis, you have to be relentlessly precise, like tightrope-walker-meets-lab-technician precise. One wrong bite and you're out.

Yes, some people drop weight quickly on keto. Most gain it back, and then some. Why? Because there's no room for birthday cake. Or balance. Or your favorite roasted carrots.

And long-term? It's hard on your organs, your breath, and your sanity.

A woman in line at Trader Joe's once said it best: "Fuck keto. I lost thirty pounds and gained back fifty-five." That's not success. That's a trap with a shiny sign.

Intermittent Fasting: Structure Without Substance

Let's be clear, there are times and places where fasting can support the body. Yet for most people using it as a weight loss tool, it's just another way to micromanage behavior without addressing the underlying issues.

If you're constantly thinking about food, shrinking the hours you're "allowed" to eat might quiet the noise. But it doesn't heal the relationship. And if the six hours in which you eat are a free-for-all, you haven't solved the problem, you've just delayed it.

Also? There's no long-term data that says this is a sustainable path to health. And if it's creating more stress than relief, your hormones are already calling BS.

Weight Loss Pills: Hope in a Bottle

There's a difference between supplements that support your biology and pills that promise to melt fat. The line gets blurred fast, especially when you're desperate.

Most fat burners and "metabolism boosters" are just expensive stimulants, diuretics, or unsubstantiated cocktails that mess with your heart rate more than your waistline. True, some ingredients, like chromium or white kidney bean extract, have evidence behind them. But no, that fizzy Alka-Seltzer-looking tablet that "melts belly fat" didn't actually win Shark Tank. It's a scam. So are most before-and-after photos. What you're seeing is lighting, angles, and sometimes Photoshop, not proof of health.

If it sounds too good to be true, it probably is.

Wellness Apps: Behavioral or Just Calorie Counting with Homework?

Noom markets itself as the anti-diet. Behavioral psychology! Lasting change! Color-coded foods! But behind the fancy UX and cheerful emails is the same old formula: eat less, move more, track everything. Only now, you get articles assigned to you like it's a nutrition-themed AP class. You're promised insight. What you get is screen fatigue, generic food traffic lights, and a sense of failure when you stop keeping up.

One user summed it up like this: "It was calorie math disguised as coaching. And it made me feel like a dropout." And for someone with actual health conditions? Some of the guidance is not just unhelpful; it might be actively harmful.

Listen, anything can work for someone…for a finite period. The goal here isn't short-term compliance. It's long-term capacity. And most of these programs aren't built for that.

The Bottom Line

The point is that none of these solutions asked you to build trust in yourself. None helped you understand your body better. None gave you tools for the messy, unpredictable reality of being human. And none of them made you the magic bullet because none of them believed you could be.

Why It's So Tempting to Keep Trying

Let's be honest: it's seductive. The shiny new plan. The before-and-after photo. The promise that this one will finally fix what the last one didn't. Especially when it's wrapped in buzzwords like "wellness," "science-backed," or "just thirty days."

When you're exhausted, overwhelmed, or quietly disappointed in yourself, the idea of starting fresh is a dopamine hit. It feels like hope.

Here's the truth: We keep reaching for external solutions because we've been taught not to trust ourselves.

You've been conditioned to believe:

- If it didn't work, it's because you didn't work hard enough
- If you stop, it means you lack discipline
- If you're struggling, you need something more rigid, more extreme, more controlled

So you start again. And again. And again.

Beth, one of my clients, put it this way: "There's a narrative that says you can't do this on your own. That you're going to fail unless you buy the product or follow the system. But that's not your voice, that's theirs." She's right. The system keeps whispering, "You can't be trusted. Let us decide for you."

And it's subtle. Over time, you internalize that voice. You start to second-guess your hunger, your preferences, your capacity. You stop listening to your body because it never seems to match what you think it "should" be saying.

But here's the thing: Your body isn't malfunctioning; your self-trust has just been overridden.

The diet industry doesn't want you to know this. Because once you stop outsourcing your power—and realize that change can come from within—you become the one thing they can't sell to: Unshakable. Self-led. Unmarketable. That's why reclaiming your agency feels so radical. Because it is.

What Actually Works (and Doesn't Require a Clean Slate)

So here's the shift: Instead of asking *What plan should I follow?* start asking, *How do I want to live?*

Because the truth is, anything can "work" in the short term. Keto can drop pounds. Fasting can suppress hunger. Apps can track every calorie you breathe near. But if you can't or don't want to live like that long-term, it's not working. It's performing.

So what does work? It's not sexy. It doesn't come with before-and-afters. But it's the stuff that actually creates sustainable health and energy.

Know Your Why

(I know this can be trite, but go with me for a minute.)

Not the surface-level stuff like "lose ten pounds" or "fit into jeans from 2012." We're talking about the real why.

Do you want more energy for your kids? To stop thinking about food 24/7? To feel like you again? To be able to get up off the toilet without assistance when you're old(er)? That's your compass. When you know why you're doing something, the noise gets quieter.

Anchor in a Few Keystone Habits

No, you don't need to overhaul your life. In fact, please don't. That's a trap. Pick two or three non-negotiables that hold you steady, especially during stressful seasons:

- A solid breakfast with protein
- Drinking water before caffeine
- Prioritizing sleep (even if it means skipping a workout, *gasp!*)
- Going for a walk after dinner
- Eating vegetables because they make you feel satisfied and alert, not because someone told you to

These don't need to be flashy. They need to be yours. And when life gets loud (hi, holidays), these are the things that help you stay grounded. Notice that I didn't say perfect.

Create Integrity With Yourself

The quickest way to erode trust in yourself is to break your promises. That doesn't mean you never skip a workout or eat dessert. It means you stop setting yourself up with unrealistic goals you can't (and don't want to) meet. Start small. Choose what you will do. Then do it. And repeat. That builds trust.

Use Accountability as Amplification, Not Obligation

You don't need someone to yell at you. You need someone who helps you stay honest, curious, and consistent. Whether it's a coach, a friend, an online community, or a text thread, find people who reflect your commitment back to you, not your guilt.

And if you're tempted by that ad, that app, that limited-time offer, ask someone you trust to reality-check it with you.

Practice Discernment

Just because it's labeled "wellness" doesn't mean it's healthful. Gluten-free milk? Vegan chicken nuggets with fifty ingredients? Soap labeled "keto"? Come on.

In the UK, Cheetos are banned. And no, not because the government is anti-snack, but because they didn't meet basic food standards. Meanwhile, here in the US, ketchup has a different ingredient list depending on where you buy it. (Spoiler: tomatoes are often not the main ingredient.)

You don't need to obsess; you simply need to stay awake. Wellness isn't about following more rules. It's about choosing with clarity. When you have a plan that's rooted in science, sanity, and self-respect, you're not tempted by shiny nonsense because you already know what works for you.

How to Spot Nonsense Before You Get Sucked In

The more you reclaim your role as the magic bullet, the more the noise will start to sound like... noise. But that doesn't mean the nonsense stops coming. Ads, influencers, fitfluencers, apps, powders, pills—it's all still coming for you. So here's how to spot the red flags before you hand over your money, time, or trust.

If it promises fast, permanent results, it's lying.

Bodies don't work like that. Behavior doesn't work like that. Biology doesn't work like that. Change takes time. It's messy. It adapts. Anything that skips those steps isn't sustainable; it's a sales pitch.

If it can't handle real life, it can't handle you.

Any plan that falls apart because you had a birthday, a vacation, a Tuesday with back-to-back meetings? That plan was never built for life. You were.

If it tells you to fear food, it's not about health.

Whether it's carbs, fat, fruit, or vegetables (yes, some plans even villainize those)—if it turns your plate into a minefield, it's not wellness. It's anxiety.

If it depends on perfection, it's a setup.

You will miss a workout. You will eat dessert. You will have days where movement means walking from your desk to the fridge and back. A system that doesn't expect that is built to make you feel like a failure. On purpose.

If it makes you feel small, restricted, or ashamed, it's not working.

Wellness isn't about shrinking. It's about expanding—your energy, your freedom, your confidence, your life. So what do you do instead? You build a BS filter. One that asks:

- Is this helping me listen to my body or silence it?
- Can I live this way forever, without resenting it?
- Would I want to model this behavior for someone I love?

If an answer is no, it's a no. Period. And if you're ever unsure? Phone a friend. Run it by someone who isn't in panic mode. Ask your coach, your community, your truth-teller circle.

Because now you know better. You know that if something doesn't work *with* your life, it won't work *for* your life. You know that most of what's marketed as wellness is just stress with better branding. You know that health isn't about shrinking—it's about strengthening.

This is about respect. For your body. Your time. Your peace. Your life. And the more you practice that respect, the more bulletproof your self-trust becomes. So the next time the industry tries to sell you a shiny new fix, you'll already know the truth:

YOU are the magic bullet. Now act like it.

2

You're Not Lazy

"*If I could just be more disciplined, I'd finally get healthy.*"

You already know the voice in your head. The one that pipes up right after the cookie, or the fries, or the skipped workout. It's the voice that says, "You blew it. You always blow it. Why can't you just have more willpower?"

And right behind that voice? The spiral that sounds something like: "Well, I already screwed up, might as well keep going." (Cue the "fuck-it" effect.) That moment when one perceived slip snowballs into the whole day (or week) unraveling.

And maybe you call it something else. Maybe it sounds like, *I'll start over tomorrow*, or *Screw it, it's been a long week, I deserve it* or *What's the point?*

Whatever form it takes, the story underneath is always the same: You think the problem is you. You think if you were just more disciplined—more committed, more motivated, more self-controlled—you wouldn't be stuck.

Let's stop right there. You don't have a willpower problem; you have a willpower misunderstanding. You've been told that willpower is a kind of moral strength. A character trait. Something you either have or don't. But what if willpower isn't a reflection of your commitment or your worth?

The truth is that willpower is real, yes, but it's not endless. It's not always available. And it's definitely not the magic key to wellness. Relying on willpower to get healthy is like relying on your phone's battery without ever charging it. Eventually, it dies. Because the battery, just like your body, doesn't have unlimited capacity.

Willpower Is Like a Muscle

Think of willpower like a muscle: it works when you use it, and it gets tired the more you demand from it. Or picture it as a cup that holds your daily capacity for things like focus, self-control, impulse management, and decision-making.

That same cup powers your ability to deal with what you're wearing that day, morning traffic, your boss's tenth email, your toddler's tantrum, your to-do list, the strategic choices on your big project, and your plan to skip the donuts.

One cup. All those demands. No wonder it feels like you're running on fumes by 3:00 p.m.

Here's where it gets real. Willpower isn't just "used up," it's chemically depleted. Glucose (yes, sugar) fuels your brain's decision-making and impulse control. When your blood sugar drops, so does your willpower. You don't just feel hangry; you are less able to make thoughtful choices.

This isn't hypothetical. In one study, judges were significantly more likely to deny parole to prisoners right before lunch, when their glucose was low. Same facts, different blood sugar, different outcomes.

It's not you. It's chemistry.

Depletion Is a Real, Daily Thing

Here's what quietly empties your willpower cup:

- **Resisting desires**: Studies show we spend up to a fifth of our waking hours fighting urges. That's three to four hours a day.
- **Making decisions**: Every yes, no, or maybe uses energy, even deciding what to eat or wear.
- **Multitasking**: Splitting your attention doesn't save time. It burns fuel.
- **Stress**: Chronic stress depletes willpower. It's both emotional and physiological.
- **Lack of sleep**: Sleep deprivation impairs your overnight willpower cup replenishment and your ability to process glucose, which means your brain has less fuel to manage cravings or think clearly.
- **Skipping meals**: Low blood sugar = low self-regulation.
- **PMS**: During the luteal phase, your body reroutes energy to the reproductive system. What's left for the rest of you? Not much. Hence, the cravings.
- **Dieting**: Restricting calories or entire food groups creates a double whammy. It depletes glucose and triggers hormonal changes that intensify cravings.

What Depletion Feels Like

The signs are sneaky but familiar:

- Overreacting to small things (the "volume" of life feels turned up)
- Indecision, especially over small stuff
- Inability to compromise (hello, tension in relationships)
- Cravings that feel louder and more urgent
- That "screw it" spiral

If any of this sounds like your Tuesday, it's not a personality flaw. It's a chemistry lesson no one ever taught.

Diets Make This Worse, Not Better

Let's zoom in on this one. Restrictive diets don't just ask you to control what you eat; they demand more willpower at the exact time your body has less of it. Remember, the brain runs on glucose. When we cut calories too hard or skip meals to be "good," we starve our brain of the fuel it needs to make thoughtful choices.

One study found that dieters drank milkshakes and ate more cookies afterward compared to those who simply hadn't eaten and then had the cookies and milkshakes placed before them. Why? Not only could they not respond to their own body's hunger and satiety cues, but their willpower was tapped.

Dieting trains you to ignore your body's cues and follow external rules instead. Over time, that erodes self-trust, the very foundation of sustainable health.

Use Willpower to Build Habits, Not to Fight Cravings

If white-knuckling worked, it would've worked by now. The goal isn't to have more willpower (although that's also helpful); it's to need less of it.

Here's the big shift: Willpower isn't your emergency brake; it's your architect. You don't need it for every decision; you do need it to build the defaults that make decisions easier. So let's talk strategy.

1. Feed Your Brain, Not Just Your Belly

- **Eat to stabilize blood sugar.** That means protein + fiber + healthful fats—not just for satiety, but for brain function.

This is why "just eat less" advice is so backwards. Low fuel = low control.

- **Focus on breakfast.** If your first meal sets off a blood sugar rollercoaster, you've already compromised your decision-making for the day. Start stable.
- **Use carbs wisely.** Your brain runs on glucose. When you starve it, it gets reactive.
- **Sleep like it's your job.** It's not a luxury. It's a glucose-regulation tool. A willpower replenisher. Less sleep = more cravings = less clarity.

In short, nutrition and sleep replenish the cup. Dieting and restriction drain it.

2. Use Willpower Upstream

Let's stop trying to summon strength at the hardest moment, like when the fries hit the table, or the cookies are in arm's reach. Use what's in your cup to set things up.

- **Pre-commit.** Brush your teeth early to signal "kitchen's closed." Pack your gym clothes the night before.
- **Make if/then plans.** *If they have brownies, I'll have fruit first. If I'm at happy hour, I'll order a club soda before deciding on food.* These become automatic decisions instead of draining ones.
- **Gamify it.** Use a tracker, a streak, a daily check-in. Tiny wins build big trust.

Remember: You're not weak in the moment. You're under-resourced. Move your effort earlier.

3. Monitor, Celebrate, Repeat

- **Write it down.** Even a simple food log gives your brain relief—less to hold, less to deplete.

- **Set small, doable goals.** "Drink water before coffee" beats "overhaul your entire food life by Friday."
- **Celebrate completions.** Cross things off. Finish things. Tiny wins refill your cup. It's biology and psychology.

Your brain trusts you when you follow through. Start small. Stay honest.

4. Lean on Accountability

- **Tell someone.** Public goals stick better than private ones. (Public doesn't have to be the entire internet; it can be one trusted friend.)
- **Track with others.** Share your steps, meals, or streaks with a buddy, coach, or app.
- **Choose your people wisely.** Some relationships refill your cup. Others poke holes in it.

Willpower is social. You're not supposed to do this alone.

5. Build Better Defaults

- **Habits don't require willpower.** That's the goal—healthful behavior on autopilot.
- **Tidy up one corner of your life.** People who made their beds daily had more self-control across the board. Why? They stopped wasting energy on daily decision-making.
- **Start with what's easiest.** Morning routine, prepping snacks, cleaning out the car—anything that says, "I follow through."

Willpower is for construction. Let your habits do the maintenance. (That's how you end up with willpower left in the cup for the unexpected, free dessert.)

6. Delay the Decision

This one's a game changer:
Instead of saying, *No*, say, *Not right now. I'll come back for that muffin if I still want it after lunch. If I want the fries later, they'll still exist.*

The delay gives your body time to refuel. It restores blood sugar, reduces urgency, and gives your rational brain a fighting chance.

7. Distract or Disrupt

You don't need to fight the craving. You need to get some distance from it.

- Go outside
- Do a breathing exercise
- Call a friend
- Put on some music and dance around the kitchen

Every time you prove to yourself that you can pause, the next time gets easier.

You Don't Need More Willpower

So let's say this plainly, one last time: Your willpower isn't broken. It's just been burned out by all the demands life throws at you. And the fix isn't "try harder" or "I just need to do it." It's "set it up sooner."

Use your willpower to set up the system so when the hard moment hits, you've already decided. This is the fundamental strategy: Use willpower to build habits, not to battle cravings.

Let the default be your safety net. Because the truth is, when you're exhausted, stressed, triggered, or tempted, you will fall back on whatever's easiest, whatever signals safety and comfort.

Your job isn't to be perfect. Your job is to make the path of least resistance work in your favor.

3

The Big C: Choosing Consistency Over Intensity

You know the feeling. It's a new year, a Monday, or maybe just a moment when you decide: "This is it. I'm doing it. For real this time." So you go hard. You clean out your kitchen, sign up for every class at the gym, maybe even commit to a no-sugar, no-wine, no-fun kind of plan. For a while, it works. You feel focused. In control. Like someone who "finally figured it out."

Then a few weeks in, maybe even just a few days, life happens. Work gets busy. You're exhausted. Someone invites you out. You skip one workout. Order takeout one night. Don't meditate. The streak breaks. And then comes the spiral. The "F-its" set in, and you're like the Tasmanian Devil cartoon character with your mouth open wide, tongue hanging out, ready to eat everything there is, and especially everything that's been on the "no-no list."

Suddenly, that initial little wobble feels like failure. The voices in your head start chirping. *See? You can't stick with anything. Why even bother? You need more willpower.*

Let me stop you right there. You didn't fail. Full. Stop.

You followed a pattern that's been drilled into us by the entire wellness-industrial complex: if you want results, you have to go hard. Hustle. Restrict. Dominate your calendar and your cravings.

Here's the truth: wellness isn't a boot camp. It's a rhythm. And rhythms—unlike bootcamps—are meant to be lived in, not suffered through.

So let's break this myth wide open. The one that says intensity is the answer. Because it's not. Not if you want to feel well, happy, and energized for more than a week.

The False Promise of Intensity

Let's give intensity its moment first, because it can be powerful.

When it comes to exercise, intensity challenges the body in ways that build strength, endurance, and capacity. That push can trigger transformation. A tough workout can feel like a reset button. A big lifestyle shift can feel like you're finally in control.

And when we're in a season of strong motivation—like after a health scare, a milestone birthday, or just feeling fed up—intensity matches our energy. It makes us feel committed. Serious. Like we're not messing around anymore.

And that's precisely the trap.

The very nature of intensity makes it hard to sustain. The more extreme the plan, the harder it is to keep showing up for it, especially when life kicks in.

Think about it: waking up early for 90-minute workouts sounds great until you're running on five hours of sleep. Cutting sugar cold turkey sounds virtuous until you're PMS-ing and your coworker brings brownies. Going all-in on a strict meal plan feels structured until you're invited to dinner and suddenly the rules don't fit.

The result? We drop off. And when we do, we blame ourselves. It's. Not. You. It's the plan.

Intensity creates spikes. Spikes aren't inherently bad; they're just not a foundation. If your health habits rely on white-knuckling through every craving, scheduling every minute, or constantly chasing "perfect," you're not building wellness. You're building burnout.

And eventually, the body—and the brain—calls it.

The Power of Consistency

Now let's talk about the unsung hero of health—consistency. I get it; it doesn't sound sexy. Consistency doesn't come with dramatic before-and-after photos or New Year's Day energy. It's not splashy. It's not extreme. Still, it's what works.

Because here's the deal: Your body doesn't respond to what you do once; it responds to what you do most of the time.

That means showing up in small, steady ways matters more than any single "perfect" day. A short walk three days a week? That moves the needle. Adding veggies to your lunch every day? That creates momentum. Getting to bed thirty minutes earlier? That impacts everything from hormones to hunger cues.

This isn't about never pushing hard. It's about choosing actions you can keep showing up for. Actions that don't require you to be in peak motivation mode to follow through.

Let me give you a metaphor. Picture two cars on an open road. (Go with me on all the car analogies throughout the book; I grew up in the suburbs of Detroit.) The first is our intensity car. It blasts down the highway at sixty miles per hour but only for three minutes. Then it stops. Then it goes again. Then stops. Again. Again. The second is the consistency car. It chugs along at 15 miles per hour, every hour, every day, no matter what.

Which one reaches the destination first? (Sincere apologies for any flashbacks to traumatic math homework with your dad.) Consistency might feel slower. Yet it gets you further. Because it doesn't rely on your best day, it meets you on your real ones.

What This Looks Like

So how do we live this? What does consistency look like in the middle of your busy, messy, full, real life? Let's start by translating this into the choices you're making every day.

Instead of…

A sixty-minute workout five days a week that leaves you sore, exhausted, and dreading the gym…

Play with this: ten to fifteen minutes of movement a couple of times a day. A walk after lunch. Some bodyweight squats before your shower. A dance break between meetings.

Instead of…

Cutting out all sugar, swearing off carbs, or going full-on detox mode…

Play with this: Add protein and fiber to every meal. Enjoy dessert with your kids and build a plate that supports your blood sugar.

Instead of…

Saying "no" to every social invite so you can "stay on track"…

Play with this: Go out, laugh, eat the fries, and notice how you feel. Then continue with your usual routine later that night, the next day, and so on. That's still forward motion.

This is the stuff that adds up.

You don't need a total overhaul. You need anchor habits that fit your life. The kind that stick around when the novelty wears off and the schedule gets weird.

And remember: perfection is not the price of progress. Showing up counts. Even if it's less than what you wanted to do. Even if it's not ideal. Because consistency isn't about doing everything—it's about doing something, regularly enough, that your body can trust you.

The Principle to Keep

If there's one thing I hope you take from this chapter, it's this: Sustainable change isn't built on how hard you can push. It's built on how often you can show up.

Consistency isn't glamorous. It doesn't come with a playlist or a countdown clock. It works, though. And when you let go of the need to do it all, perfectly, all the time, you create space to do the things that matter, often enough to feel better.

Intensity has its place. It can shake things up, add variety, or match a moment of big motivation. It's just not the foundation. It's the spice, not the main dish.

So the next time you catch yourself feeling behind or not "doing enough," ask, *Am I expecting myself to be intense and consistent at the same time?*

Because that's a tough road to run. Instead, choose consistency, done your way. In your real life. On your terms. Small steps, in the same direction, over time, lead to huge distances.

4

Your Genes Are Not the Boss of You

You've probably said it, or at least thought it, *It's in my genes*. It's one of those phrases we use that feels like a full stop. We say it to explain why our cravings are so intense, why the weight won't budge, why our cholesterol is high, and why certain health issues seem to follow us no matter what we do. And for a long time, we were taught that was the end of the story.

What if it's not? Yes, genes are important. They're the blueprint for how our bodies are built and how they function. But—and this is a big but—they're not the boss of you.

Somewhere along the way, genes became this looming, deterministic explanation for everything from weight gain to cravings to why your entire family hates cilantro. And while genetics does play a role, it's not the final word. And it turns out, it's a lot more like drafting the outline than writing the entire story.

Genetics 101

Genes are segments of DNA, tiny sequences that tell our bodies how to build and function. Think of them like a blueprint: they lay out the possibilities. Your height, your eye color, and whether your earlobes are attached or not. Additionally, factors such as how your body processes sugar, how well it responds to nutrition and movement, and even your tendency to crave salt or sweets are also considered.

That field of study—how traits get passed from generation to generation—is called "genetics." And sure, some of that might explain why you and your sibling both reach for chips when stressed, or why heart disease shows up in your family tree.

But here's where we need to get clear: Family history and genetics are NOT the same thing. It's easy to say, "Oh, diabetes runs in my family," and assume it's purely genetic. What everyone overlooks is that families don't just share genes; they share lifestyle. They share habits, routines, food culture, stress patterns, sleep schedules, and stories about what health "should" look like. So what we call "family history" is often as much about environment and behavior as it is about biology. Remember the old nature vs. nurture debate? It belongs here, too.

And this is an incredible thing. Because while you can't exactly go back and edit your DNA, what you can influence is how that DNA expresses.

How Epigenetics Changes the Story

So you've got your genetic blueprint. Guess what? Blueprints don't build houses. People do.

That's where epigenetics comes in. It's the study of how your behaviors and environment influence the way your genes show up. In other words, just because a gene can express a certain trait doesn't mean it will. A lot of that depends on how you're living your life.

Here's how I like to think of it. Make a fist with one hand. That's your gene. Now, take your other hand and wrap it around the fist. That's epigenetics. It's everything surrounding your gene: what you eat, how you sleep, how much stress you're under, how active you are, what you're exposed to in your environment.

And just like a hand can loosen or tighten its grip, epigenetics can dial up or dial down the expression of that gene. It's like a volume knob. The gene is still there, but how loudly it plays is flexible.

This is the difference between predisposition and destiny. You might be wired to gain weight more easily, to have stronger cravings, or to develop insulin resistance. Those are possibilities, not guarantees.

That's a powerful shift. It means you're not a prisoner of your DNA. You're the DJ. You can adjust the volume up or down based on what you do every day.

What Your DNA Doesn't Decide

Years ago, I worked with a DNA test that analyzed your genes and gave lifestyle recommendations based on them. One part of the report was an "obesity score"—a number from 0 to 10 indicating your genetic propensity for obesity.

My score? 8.6 out of 10. That number hit me hard. It explained so much. It wasn't just in my head when I felt like I could breathe and gain weight.

And I wasn't alone. One of my mentors, a former professional football player with a body that looked nothing like mine, had a score of 8.2. Different bodies, similar predisposition—and of the two of us, I was more likely to look like an offensive lineman.

Here's what that taught me:

1. I wasn't imagining it. Some of us do have more stacked against us.

2. If I didn't do the things I do—manage stress, prioritize sleep, eat with intention, move regularly—my health would be completely different.

That's the thing, right? My genes didn't make the decision; my habits did (and do).

So no, you're not doomed. Even if your family tree is full of heart disease or your 23andMe report feels like a list of landmines, you still have power. Your blueprint may be set, but what you build from it? That's in your hands.

What Impacts Gene Expression

This is where epigenetics comes in, as the biological mechanism that responds to those habits. It's how your body interprets and expresses your DNA based on what it's exposed to day after day. Another visual for you: think of a marionette, a puppet with strings (O.G. Pinocchio style). Your DNA are the strings, your epigenetics are the hand that pulls each string to move the puppet.

Research has identified a handful of key lifestyle and environmental factors that influence gene expression through epigenetic pathways. And spoiler alert: You already know most of them. Now, instead of hearing them as generic "healthy habits," you can understand them as levers—real, proven influences on how your genes behave.

Here's what we're talking about:

- Nutrition
- Obesity
- Physical activity
- Tobacco use
- Alcohol consumption
- Environmental toxins
- Psychological stress
- Sleep quality and disruption (like working night shifts)

These aren't just wellness buzzwords. They're the inputs your body is constantly responding to at a genetic level. And while you can't rewrite the DNA itself, you *can* reshape the way it shows up in your life.

Let's be clear: lifestyle doesn't change your genes. You can't swap them out like batteries. But you can change how much they influence you. That volume knob metaphor? This is where it matters. Daily choices dial things up or down over time.

So that sugar craving you can't shake? That weight that won't budge even when you're "doing everything right"? It may have a genetic component. But how much power it has in your life isn't fixed.

And this is where you get to step in, not with a 30-day plan or a detox tea, but with real, sustainable shifts that add up.

Let me give you a real-life example. Bonnie came to me early last year, frustrated and frankly, skeptical. She told me her CRP, a marker of inflammation in the body, was always high and so was her cholesterol. Same with her siblings. "It's in our genes," she said. "No matter what I do, nothing changes."

Sound familiar? She joined my 12-week program in late January. By the halfway point, she had a new doctor who ran updated bloodwork.

Here's what we found:

- Her CRP dropped almost a whole point and was now just a hair outside the optimal range
- Total cholesterol was down more than 50 points
- HDL (the "good" cholesterol) went up
- LDL dropped by over 40 points
- Triglycerides were down more than 25 points
- And non-HDL cholesterol dropped nearly 50 points

How did we do it? We adjusted her nutrition, looked at sleep and stress, added a few targeted supplements, and started working toward more consistent movement. That's it. No extremes. No detoxes. No tracking every bite.

She was shocked. I wasn't. Because when we change the environment around our genes—how we eat, sleep, move, and manage stress—our bodies respond. Sometimes faster than we expect.

The Catch (and the Hope)

Now, before we all run off to overhaul our lives, let's get honest. Epigenetics isn't magic. It doesn't work because you ate one salad or took a walk once last week. These shifts take time. And more than that, they take consistency. (There's that word again.)

I know, that's not a sexy answer. It is the true one, though. The changes you make today, tomorrow, and next week all stack up. Your genes respond not to what you do occasionally, but to what you do regularly. That doesn't mean you have to be perfect. It means you have to show up. More often than not.

So if you've been feeling stuck or overwhelmed, hear this: You don't have to do everything. You just have to do something and keep doing it. Manage stress. Prioritize sleep. Move your body. Eat quality food. Repeat.

These are not revolutionary ideas, and that's precisely the point. You don't need a revolutionary solution. You need a reliable one.

5

There's a Problem with Your Yardstick

How do you know if something's working for you?

For most of us, the answer depends on numbers: step counts, calorie goals, minutes exercised, pounds lost, and inches measured. We've been taught to treat these numbers as truth, as gospel. And when we fall short, we blame ourselves. Worse? Sometimes we hit the numbers, and yet we still don't feel any better, still don't see the change we were promised.

What if the problem isn't you? What if it's the measuring stick? This is why I preach guidelines, not gospel.

If you've listened to my podcast, you've probably heard me say that before. And I'll keep saying it because it's the anchor I come back to with every client, every conversation, every time we get caught in the loop of "not doing it right." We've been taught to measure progress with someone else's ruler. But when the metric is off, the message is too.

So let's back up. What if you started measuring your choices not by the scale, calories, rules, or your Apple Watch, but by something more helpful and true for you?

Like:

- How does my body feel physically?
- Did I sleep well last night?
- Do I have energy?
- Did that meal satisfy me or send me scavenging an hour later?
- Am I feeling stronger, clearer, more confident?

Paying attention to our minds and bodies is how we begin practicing discernment. And it's one of the most powerful tools you have. Because the truth is, no one needs more rules. We all just need to develop a better yardstick.

Rewriting the Workout Yardstick

If you didn't close your rings, did it even count?

Let's talk about exercise, the yardstick most of us learned to fear. We've been taught to measure workouts with intensity, duration, or how drenched in sweat we end up. Ten thousand steps. A million reps. Sixty minutes. Heart rate zones. Calories burned. Green circles closed. If you didn't hit those, what was the point, right?

Wrong. That's hustle culture disguised as health. (*Gulp.* Maybe read that again.)

Here's what I see all the time: someone moves their body, stretches, walks, even dances a little while folding laundry, and then dismisses it as "not a real workout." Why? Because it didn't check the box. It wasn't long enough. It didn't leave them gasping on the floor. And that box? That's someone else's box. You don't have to live inside it.

Let me ask you this: Did you move your body today? If yes, it counts.

When the measure is moving your body today, we open the door to consistency. And consistency, not intensity, is what improves your health over time. It also builds self-trust, which, as I've mentioned, is critical for true, sustainable wellness.

Have you heard people say "sitting is the new smoking"? It's because it's the thing we're doing that we don't realize is slowly killing us. It's not human to sit all day. In response to that, we have this wild workout expectation. To which I also say, sitting all day and going berserk for an hour is also not human. In fact, it's just as "not human" as sitting all day. What is human? Regular bouts of moving your body in various ways throughout the day.

Now, does this mean your Apple Watch is evil? No. It can be a helpful tool if *you* are the one defining success. If we use it as a tool to see our own progress, it can be helpful. Yet when your metrics start to come with judgment, shame, or competition (hello, social tracking apps), it's time to reassess. Are your devices keeping you accountable, or are they keeping you anxious, feeling "not enough"? For some of us, they're helpful. For others, not so much.

And let's not forget, every body is different. What feels empowering in your thirties might feel punishing in your fifties. What used to be motivating might now feel like a mental hurdle. And that's okay. In fact, it is totally natural. Our bodies were built to move, so if you're moving in a way that feels supportive for your body, congratulations, friend. That's the whole point.

So here's a better workout yardstick:

- Did I move today?
- Did I feel powerful doing it?
- Did it support my energy, my joints, my mood?

If yes, it counts. Even if it was a ten-minute walk or a walk to the mailbox. Even if it was gentle stretching while binge-watching your favorite show.

Food Math Fails

Because Twix and eggplant are not created equal.

Brace yourself, I'm about to come for one of wellness and diet culture's most sacred cows.

Calories are a terrible yardstick.

There, I said it. Now, before anyone lights the torches, hear me out. I'm not saying calories don't exist. I'm saying the way we use them—as the only or primary measure of what and how much to eat—is wildly misleading. And honestly? It's doing more harm than good.

We've been told over and over: eat fewer calories than you burn, and the weight will come off. That assumes all calories are equal. And they're not. You know this, too (even without tons of research or a biology or nutrition degree). 1,200 calories of Twix ≠ 1,200 calories of eggplant.

(Also, I wouldn't recommend either of those. Not to mention, 1,200 calories? That's what toddlers eat. Unless you're a very small child or a houseplant, that number is not your benchmark.)

Food isn't just math: it's chemistry. It's protein, fiber, quality fats, vitamins, minerals, and phytonutrients. It's the stuff your cells use to build neurotransmitters (think mood), hormones, repair tissue, regulate blood sugar, power your brain, support your immune system—all of it. A calorie tells you nothing about any of that. It's like judging a book by the number of pages instead of what's on each page.

The same goes for the "Percent Daily Value" on nutrition labels. Those numbers were designed for the military in the early 1930s, leading up to World War II, to make sure soldiers didn't develop rickets and scurvy, not to optimize your energy, immunity, or brain function. They made their way to your food label in the 1970s, yet were still based on the minimum needed to avoid illness, not the ideal for feeling and living well. And let's be honest: they weren't exactly tested on multitasking, menstruating, child-bearing, sleep-deprived women who keep everyone fed and alive. So if you've ever seen 25 percent of your fat for the day in two tablespoons of peanut butter and panicked—don't. That label isn't your health destiny. It's a wartime survival guide that got grandfathered into your pantry.

And then there are the diet tribes: keto, paleo, Whole30, insert-trademarked-plan here. These aren't inherently evil. But when we treat their food lists like gospel, we get stuck in binary thinking: this food is clean, that one is dirty. This one is allowed. That one is cheating. And suddenly we're not eating, we're performing.

Let me offer a better barometer—nutrition. What's the quality of the food you're eating? Is it nutrient-dense? Does it include fiber, protein, and quality fat to keep you full and fueled? Is it colorful? (Yes, literal color—the more natural variety, the better.) Is it satisfying, or are you raiding the pantry twenty minutes after your lunch?

That's the stuff that matters. That's what fuels your body and your life. So no, I don't care how many calories are in your avocado. I care how it makes you feel because that is information worth measuring.

And for what it's worth, for all the people who made it this far and are still skeptical, holding onto their calorie and macro tracking apps, I promise you the calories will take care of themselves when we eat for nutrition. Your body can self-regulate blueberries. It cannot self-regulate Skittles. After eighteen years of coaching others (as of 2025), I see it every time. I promise you. The calories will take care of themselves.

Portion Distortion

If you're measuring your food by someone else's appetite, we've got a problem.

Portion size is one of those areas where many of us tend to spiral. We don't just look at what's on our plate. We look at what's on everyone else's. Your partner eats as much as you, so you wonder if you're overeating. Your friend eats half as much, so you feel guilty for finishing your meal.

Let me say this clearly: What someone else eats is not a valid yardstick for what you need. Your body isn't theirs. Your metabolism isn't theirs. Your day, your muscle mass, your stress, your hormones—they're all different. So the fact that your partner can crush a burger and fries and still want dessert? Not your business. Not your benchmark.

And don't even get me started on restaurants. Most of them serve portions that are two to three times what a body needs. That doesn't mean you can't enjoy a meal out. It just means you don't have to treat their serving size as a prescription (hello, clean plate club members). You also don't have to automatically cut it in half and then beat yourself up for wanting more than half.

If you're looking for a portion guide that respects your body, here's my favorite: your hands.

- Protein? One hand (a full hand at a meal, the palm at a snack).
- Leafy greens? Two big handfuls.
- Whole grains? One fist.
- Fruit and starchy veg? One cupped handful.
- Quality fats? Your thumb.

Why your hands? Because they scale with your body. They're portable. And unlike measuring cups or a food scale, they don't make you feel like you're prepping for a lab experiment instead of lunch.

Even better? Tune in to hunger. And I don't mean emotional hunger—I mean that honest, stomach-growling, "would I eat broccoli right now?" kind of hunger. If the only thing that sounds good is Reese's pieces, you might be craving comfort, not calories. (That's not a crime, by the way. It's just helpful to recognize the difference.)

So next time you catch yourself scanning someone else's plate, remember: Your body, your fuel, is not a group project. You don't need to match your portions to anyone else's pace, preference, or plate size. You need to feed *yourself*.

Choice, Not Cheating

You didn't "cheat;" you ate a cookie.

Let's clear something up once and for all: Food is not a morality test. There is no such thing as "being bad" because you had a slice of cake. You're not "cheating" because you ate bread. You didn't "fall off the wagon;" you just ate something.

The moralization of food choices is one of the most damaging yardsticks in wellness culture. As if the contents of your plate say anything about your worth or your character. They don't.

So let's reframe: every bite you take is a choice. That's it. Not a sin. Not a failure. A choice. And you get to make it based on how it aligns with your goals, your energy, your joy, and your body.

There's real power in that. When you take the judgment out of eating, you give yourself space to make intentional decisions instead of reactionary ones. So maybe you ask:

- Does this move me closer to how I want to feel?
- Is this something I'm choosing because I genuinely want it or because I feel stressed, tired, or pressured?
- Can I enjoy this without making it mean I've blown everything?

Because let me tell you: a cookie doesn't cancel your progress. Guilt might. Shame can. That spiral where one "off" moment turns into a week (or month or year) of giving up and needing to "start over"? That's what sets you back.

And while it sounds like I'm only talking about language, the words we use reflect our mindset. When you shift from "I'm on a diet" to "this is my nutrition," you start seeing food as fuel, not punishment. You stop treating eating like a tightrope walk and start living like a person.

Food isn't a test. You don't need to pass or fail it. You just need to pay attention, make conscious choices, and let go of the idea that some foods are "bad" while others are "good."

So next time you catch yourself thinking *I was bad* or *I can't have that*, take a breath and ask, *What am I actually measuring here?* Because odds are, you're using someone else's broken yardstick, and it's time to put it down.

BMI is B.S. (and the Scale's Not Much Better)

If the scale is your only yardstick, you're missing the whole picture.

For many people, the scale has become the ultimate truth-teller. We step on it, hoping for validation, dreading disappointment, and measuring our entire effort (not to mention self-worth) by whatever it flashes back at us.

Here's the thing: The scale is not a health detector; it's a snapshot of gravity.

That number includes your bones, organs, water, muscle, fat, brain, hair gel, breakfast—you get the point. It's everything. And it doesn't distinguish between any of it. You could gain five pounds of muscle and lose five pounds of fat, and the scale wouldn't budge. Your health though? Dramatically improved. And for what it's worth, there are zero (ZERO!) diseases that exist only in bigger bodies.

So why are we letting it be the judge and jury? Worse, some weight-loss programs actively discourage strength training before weigh-ins because building muscle might make the number go up, even if you're genuinely getting healthier. That's how broken our metrics have become: they're designed to chase optics, not outcomes.

And then there's BMI, which stands for Body Mass Index but might as well be renamed Blatantly Misleading Indicator. It was created in the 1800s (yes, eighteen) to study population trends, not individuals. It doesn't account for body composition, frame, age, or muscle mass. According to BMI, Dwayne "The Rock" Johnson is obese. Enough said.

If our goal is health—not just shrinking ourselves—then we need better benchmarks. Body composition is one. Use a tape measure. Track your body fat percentage over time. Look at how your clothes fit, how your energy feels, how you sleep, and how your joints move.

There are even home scales that estimate body fat percentage. Are they perfect? No. But if you use the same one consistently and under the same conditions (same time of day, clothes, similar hydration), you'll start to see trends, and trends are more useful than snapshots.

The key here? Context. Not just data, but what the data means.

Because if your body fat is going down and your energy is going up, but the scale hasn't moved? That's still a win. If you're lifting more, sleeping better, or waking up without pain? That's health. That's progress. The scale just isn't smart enough to see it (yet).

So let's stop pretending one number can tell the whole story. You are not your weight. And you are definitely not your BMI.

Metrics That Matter

Here's the reframe wellness culture desperately needs: Progress is not a number; it's a feeling. And yet, most of us were taught to chase a very narrow definition of success: lower weight, smaller pants, more willpower. In reality, those aren't the wins that change your life.

Let me ask you:

- Do you get out of bed without aching?
- Are your moods more stable?
- Are your cravings less chaotic?
- Are you eating meals and feeling satisfied instead of always feeling peckish?
- Do you feel less guilt around food—or less like you're constantly starting over?

Because that is real progress. That's the stuff that makes life feel doable again.

One of my clients made two small nutrition shifts in one week. That's it, just two tweaks. And within days, she was waking up without pain for the first time in years. She couldn't even remember what that felt like. Now, no scale in the world could capture that transformation. But she could feel it. And that's what matters.

We have to stop confusing "easy in the moment" with "effective in the long run." Sure, grabbing a candy bar while on the road might feel like a quick fix, but if it comes with a week of guilt and mental chatter, is it really easier? What if we started measuring peace instead of perfection? And what if we measured ease by how confidently we move through our day, not by how convenient it is to beat ourselves up?

Comparison makes all of this harder. We look at what other people eat, how fast they "bounce back," what they post, what they wear—and make it mean something about us. But that's apples and oranges. Their yardstick is not your yardstick. And honestly, it might not be working for them either.

So let's create some new metrics, ones that reflect health, not hustle:

- Quality of sleep
- Resilience to stress
- Steady energy
- Clear thinking
- Confidence in yourself and your choices
- Joy around food

If your yardstick isn't measuring those things, it might be time to retire it. The goal isn't to perform health, but to feel well in your body, your mind, and your everyday life.

Pick a New Yardstick

If you've ever felt like you were doing everything "right" and still not getting anywhere, hear this: you haven't failed. Your yardstick has. You've been measuring success with tools that were never built for you, tools designed to sell plans, push products, or track populations, not support your unique body and life. Of course, it hasn't worked. Of course, you're tired. It's exhausting to chase goals that aren't your own.

Here's the good news: you get to pick a new yardstick. You get to define what progress means. You get to decide what matters. You get to stop chasing perfection and start choosing metrics that reflect your actual goals, not someone else's expectations.

So take a moment. Ask yourself:

- How do I want to feel?
- What would success look like if no one else were watching?
- What matters more to me: the number on the scale, or the energy to play with my kids? The inches on my waist, or the fact that I woke up pain-free for the first time in months?

This is your permission slip to recalibrate. To swap judgment for curiosity. To choose metrics that tell the truth about what matters to you.

6

Top 5 Tips for Digesting Nutrition News

Practicing discernment when the noise breaks through.

You don't need a PhD to make smart choices about your health. Except in today's wellness world, it can feel like you do. One day, red wine is healthy for your heart. The next, even a sip raises your blood pressure. Dairy causes inflammation—unless it's in ice cream, then it's suddenly heart-healthy (Happy National Ice Cream Day, right?).

If you've ever read a headline and thought, *Wait, what am I supposed to eat now?*—you're not alone. And more importantly, you're not crazy. The system is chaotic by design. Clicks get prioritized over clarity. Sensation over science. And wellness advice? It's been spun, stretched, and sold so many times that it's almost impossible to recognize what's actually helpful. Because you don't need more noise, you need a filter.

These are the five questions I ask any time I see a new nutrition claim, trend, or "hot tip." They've helped me avoid shiny-object syndrome, protect my energy, and stay grounded in what truly matters. My clients use them. My podcast guests talk about them. And after today, you'll have them too.

I call them my "Top 5 Tips for Digesting Nutrition News." (Yes, the pun is intentional.) But really? They're a crash course in wellness discernment, aka your secret weapon for cutting through the noise and reclaiming your focus.

5. Sources and Benefactors

Follow the money. And the microphone.

Let's start where we wish every headline would—with the question, "Who's behind this?" Because whether it's a study, an article, a viral TikTok, or a doctor on morning TV, you have to ask: Who funded this? Who benefits from my believing it?

We're not talking conspiracy theory. We're talking basic media literacy. Just like in food, ingredients matter, and so do incentives.

Let's say you read a headline that says, "New research shows cheese improves metabolic health." Okay, sounds delicious. But was that research funded by an independent institution? Or by the dairy board? (It's a real thing.) Was it published in a peer-reviewed journal? Or summarized in a press release sent to every morning show producer in the country?

Here's the thing: Industry-funded research isn't inherently unhelpful. Sometimes, the only people willing to pay for a study are the ones who stand to gain from it. That doesn't make the science automatically wrong; it just means we need to read it with context.

The same goes for media outlets. If an article is quoting experts, who are they? Are they the ones who ran the study, or independent scientists reviewing it? Is the outlet itself tied to any industry interests? (A quick look at the About Us page can tell you a lot.)

There's also something called indication drift, which is when research on one population gets used to justify treatment in a totally different one. For example, a drug studied in high-risk, unvaccinated individuals gets marketed to everyone. Or a diet that showed benefits for epileptic children suddenly becomes a weight-loss plan for adults (lean in so I can whisper this—it's called keto). The application has drifted far from the evidence.

Nutrition is especially vulnerable to this. Many fad diets started from research that had a very specific scope, but marketing doesn't care about nuance. Marketing cares about momentum.

This is why your first filter isn't, *Is this true?* It's, *Who said this, and what are they standing to gain?* You don't have to throw out every headline. You do get to ask better questions. And those questions protect your energy, your time, and your trust in your own decisions.

4. Not All Science Is Equal

Because "a study said" is not the same as "this is true."

Let me say this clearly: science matters. But not all science is created equal. What's more, science, by definition, can change. It's not a one-and-done, tick-the-box approach; we are always learning more.

If that sounds confusing or even sacrilegious, stay with me, because this is one of the most significant sources of wellness whiplash. A new headline drops. It references a study. Everyone panics or pivots. And next thing you know, someone's telling you that blueberries prevent Alzheimer's—because a study said so. (It didn't; I made this up for demonstration purposes.)

But what kind of study? Here's a quick cheat sheet:

At the bottom of the credibility ladder:

- A case study is essentially one person's experience. Compelling, sure—especially when you're the "n"—but still anecdotal. Great for learning your own patterns, risky when we assume N = 1 means "this works for everyone."
- Cell culture studies look at how compounds interact with isolated cells in a lab. Useful for early clues, but potentially not for real-life guidance.
- Animal studies are the next step up. Controlled but not human, and often tested in extreme doses to study toxicity.

Then, better:

- Epidemiological studies track large groups of people over time to spot patterns. These are often used in nutrition research, but they rely heavily on self-reported data. That means someone trying to remember what they ate last Tuesday, or last year. Still helpful. Still flawed.

The gold standard:

- Randomized Controlled Trials (RCTs). These divide people into groups randomly, test an intervention, and compare outcomes. They're expensive, time-consuming, and rare in nutrition, but when they're done well, they give us the clearest picture.

So if you're reading a headline that says, "New Study Shows..."—your follow-up question isn't *What does it say?* It's, *What kind of study is this? How was it done? And who was it done on?*

Because research in young, healthy men doesn't always translate to women in menopause. Or people with autoimmune conditions. Or literally any other human experience. Yet we apply findings broadly, often based on a single, small, preliminary study. That's how we get dietary trends like intermittent fasting or keto being marketed as one-size-fits-all.

Also? Peer review matters. Some of the splashiest "new science" isn't even published yet. It's what's called a preprint, meaning other experts haven't vetted it. This doesn't mean it's garbage. It means it's not ready to be gospel.

And lastly: if the article doesn't link to the actual study? That's your red flag. (Or at least a pink one.)

3. Be Careful of Your Own Bias

Yes, even your love for red wine has an agenda.

Most of us aren't starting from neutral when we read a headline. We're hoping it confirms what we already want to believe. "Oh, look, a Harvard study says ice cream might be good for your heart? Excellent. That's the kind of science I believe in."

This isn't a flaw. It's human nature. Our brains are wired for confirmation bias—the tendency to seek out, remember, and interpret information in a way that supports our existing beliefs. It's how we make sense of the world. But when it comes to wellness, it can backfire.

Because if you've already decided intermittent fasting is amazing, you'll skip past the nuance in a study that questions it. And if you've had a bad experience with medication, you might overlook solid science supporting its use in a different context. Our own preferences shape what feels true.

On a larger scale, our beliefs about food, medicine, and even movement get braided into our identity. "I don't take drugs." "I'm plant-based." "I'm a clean eater." These might start as preferences, but over time, they can harden into tribal alliances. And then, even quality research can feel threatening if it challenges our camp.

The trick isn't to remove all bias. That's impossible. But you can name it.

Pause and ask:

- "Am I drawn to this article because it reinforces what I want to believe?"
- "If this study said the opposite, would I trust it as much?"
- "What am I afraid might be true here and why?"

This is what I mean when I say true wellness starts with discernment. You don't need to abandon your beliefs. You just need to stay curious. Curiosity is the antidote to both fear and fanaticism.

2. Use Your Spidey Sense and Your Common Sense

Because not every headline deserves your cortisol.

You know that tingling feeling when something just doesn't sit right? That's your Spidey sense. (Yes, we're going full super-hero here. Cape optional.) Your Spidey sense is that internal nudge that says, "Huh, really?" when you read headlines like:

"Broccoli Linked to Cancer Risk."
"Experts Say Ice Cream May Be Good for Your Heart."
"The #1 Food That Will Destroy Your Gut."
"You'll Only Learn This Here, The Thing No One Else is Telling You."

It isn't your cynicism rearing its ugly head; it's your intuition flagging something as off. And you've been around long enough to know that nuance rarely fits in a headline. And usually? The truth is more boring than dramatic.

So when your Spidey sense lights up, pair it with another superpower—common sense.

For example, if a headline says something like "Even one glass of wine raises blood pressure," ask:

- Compared to what baseline?
- Over what period?
- In what population?
- And was the increase clinically significant or just statistically measurable?

Sometimes these articles point to a real association. And here's the key distinction: Correlation is not causation. Just because A and B show up together doesn't mean A caused B. Maybe the people drinking that daily glass of wine were also managing chronic stress, getting poor sleep, or eating out every night. Or maybe they were drinking the wine because of the stress, which would raise blood pressure anyway. The headline doesn't tell you that. You have to read between the lines.

And sometimes? The dose makes the poison.

That study that claims something is toxic? It might be based on absurd quantities that have zero relevance to real life. Like consuming 15 pounds of sweet potatoes a day. Or injecting isolated compounds into rats at 10,000 times the amount you'd ever get from food. Your common sense knows this. Let it speak.

And if you're still unsure, here's a helpful test: Would your grandma raise an eyebrow? Would your best friend say, "Wait, what?" That's your cue to slow down, take a breath, and check your sources. Let your Spidey sense be the alert system. Let your common sense be the filter. Together, they keep you grounded and protect you from unnecessary food anxiety.

1. Put On Your Wonder Woman Bangles

Deflect the noise. Protect your focus. Keep moving forward.

You remember Wonder Woman, right? Golden cuffs. Hair blowing in slow motion. Deflecting bullets like, "Not today, chaos." That's the energy we need when it comes to health news. Because in today's world, the bullets are flying.

"Top 5 Superfoods for Brain Health!"
"The One Food You Should NEVER Eat Again!"
"Experts Say THIS Is the Secret to Longevity!"

It's all urgency. All capital letters. All exclamation points. And if you're not careful, it'll hijack your brain (and your grocery cart) before you've even finished your coffee.

But most of these headlines don't matter. They're not written to inform you. They're written to activate your fear, your guilt, your dopamine. It's clickbait disguised as credibility. And the more overwhelmed you feel, the more likely you are to reach for a quick fix.

That's why your Wonder Woman bangles are so important. They're the metaphorical armor you can put on whenever you need to filter the noise and stay focused on what truly works for you.

Let's name some of those things, shall we?

- More vegetables
- More whole foods
- Less added sugar
- Less refined, ultra-processed stuff
- Moving your body in ways that feel supportive
- Getting enough sleep
- Drinking water
- Managing stress (or at least naming it)
- Consistency (aka small things, on repeat)

Not sexy. Not headline-worthy. Wildly effective. So when you hear about a new miracle food or a scary new risk or the diet trend everyone's "finally talking about"—pause. Tap your bangles. Ask:

- "Does this support what I already know works for me?"
- "Is this aligned with the fundamentals, or is it a shiny object?"
- "Who's saying this, and what are they trying to sell me?"

And then, if you're still curious? Cool. You can dig deeper, from a place of grounded clarity, not from fear or FOMO. Also, let's be real: sometimes the noise doesn't come from the internet. It comes from your group chat. Or your mom. Or your coworker who read a thing on Reddit and is now convinced *everyone* should be drinking celery juice at sunrise.

You can smile. You can be curious. And you can still choose what works for you.

PART II

Build Your Biostack

7

Biostack Over Biohack

L et's talk about a word that's everywhere in wellness right now: biohacking. Maybe you've seen it in videos of cold plunges or high-tech wearables promising to upgrade your sleep, energy, or metabolism. The promise? A shortcut to better energy, faster metabolism, better sleep—all without changing much in your life. Sounds impressive until you realize it's mostly smoke and mirrors.

Here's the problem: biohacks are designed to give you a slight edge (like 10 percent), and when everything else is already working, that's tremendous! They assume you're functioning at 90 percent, and you're pushing for 100. But most of us aren't anywhere near that (hard reality). We're juggling all the balls of staying on top of work, taking care of our families, managing stress, and maybe, if we're lucky, fitting in a vegetable or two.

When we grab a "hack" hoping it'll fix things, we're skipping the stuff that genuinely moves the needle. It's like putting racing tires on a car that hasn't had an oil change since 2019. Cool feature. Wrong problem.

You've been sold solutions without the whole picture and definitely without context. So while you're trying to survive on caffeine and cortisol, the wellness world is out here handing you cold plunges and chlorophyll drops.

So before you reach for a hack, let's ask a better question: What would it look like to build a system that supports your health every single day without needing to be extreme, expensive, or exhausting? That's where biostacking comes in.

A 10 Percent Bump Won't Cut It

A biohack, by definition, is meant to give you a 10 percent bump. So if your sleep is solid, your digestion's on point, your stress isn't running the show, and you wake up with real energy—sure, go ahead and try the cryotherapy or invest in a $700 infrared sauna blanket. You're ready for the bonus upgrade. For most people? That's not reality.

Ask yourself:

- Do you wake up feeling rested, or do you need coffee to feel human?
- Do you fall asleep easily and stay asleep?
- Are your energy and mood stable throughout the day or do you crash by 3:00 p.m.?
- Do you get sick easily?
- Is your digestion predictable, your stress manageable, your body composition in a place that feels sustainable to you, and equates to your desired health outcomes?

If the answer to most of those is "uh, not really," you're not alone. And you're not failing. You're also not yet in a place where a biohack will have much of an impact. Because biologically, your systems are still playing catch-up.

Statistically, over 85 percent of the US population is metabolically unwell, meaning most of us are not functioning at 90 percent; maybe we're at 50 percent or 60 percent. Now that biohack brings us to 55 percent or 65 percent. Noticeable difference? Not sure.

When the body is under stress (whether that's from poor sleep, nutrient deficiencies, blood sugar swings, inflammation, or emotional overload), it downregulates non-essential functions to preserve energy. That means even if you give it a compelling input, like a cold plunge or an NAD supplement, it might not be able to use it the way you hoped. The body's busy keeping the lights on.

I see it with clients all the time: people layering on supplements or health gadgets while skipping breakfast, "hydrating" with lattes, and pushing through exhaustion. And then they wonder why they don't feel better, why they can't lose weight, why their hormones look like they're menopausal in their mid-thirties.

Biostacking is Your Foundation

Here's the good news: if biohacks are the icing, biostacks are the cake. Biostacking involves doing small, foundational things consistently, and across the areas that run your body. Think of it as building your health like you'd build muscle: one rep, one habit, one day at a time.

I think about it in seven categories. These are the areas that, when supported, create the baseline your body needs to function, heal, and feel better.

1. **Food and Fuel**

   If you listen to my podcast or are a past client, you've heard me say it (and you're shocked this is only its first appearance in the book): Protein and fiber in every meal make removing fat no big deal. Start your day with 30 to 40 grams of protein. Stack in vegetables; 8 to 12 servings over the course of the day isn't excessive. (It is a lot of food; you won't be hungry). Add 2 to 4 servings of quality fats. Keep grains and starches smart and supportive. These aren't diet rules, they're fuel choices that work with your biology, not against it.

2. **Hydration**
   Water is a delivery system. If you're dehydrated, nothing else functions well. A general goal is half your body weight in ounces per day. Add a pinch of quality sea salt for minerals, or throw in frozen fruit to make it taste good. Carry the bottle. Set an alarm (or twelve). Make it happen.

3. **Activity**
   Movement doesn't require a gym membership or a 6:00 a.m. bootcamp. It requires frequency. Ten squats in the kitchen. A walk after eating lunch. Some resistance bands next to your desk. This isn't about earning your food; it's about building your metabolism and longevity. (Muscle is expensive tissue. You have to work for it.)

4. **Sleep**
   The quality of your day starts the night before. Stack your sleep by getting morning light, cutting off food a few hours before bed, dimming overhead lights, and, yes, putting the phone down. (I know. That one's hard. I'm working on it too.)

5. **Stress**
   You're not going to eliminate stress. That's not the goal. The goal is to give your body tools to handle it: breathing before meals, five quiet minutes between calls, or a walk instead of scrolling. Your nervous system will thank you.

6. **Mindset**

This one's sneaky. Are you saying to yourself (or aloud), *I have to work out*. Or *I get to move*? Are you telling yourself you're lazy, or reminding yourself you're learning? Words matter. Play matters. Fun matters. You're not a robot, you're a person. Treat yourself like one.

And listen, we tackled this one hard back in Part 1 for a reason. Mindset shapes how you approach everything else. If you notice yourself slipping into all-or-nothing thinking or beating yourself up, go back and re-read those chapters. This work is nuanced and layered, and it takes time (and lots of reinforcement). That's not a flaw in you; that's just how brains work.

7. **Connection**

Hug your kid. Hold your partner's hand. Text a friend who gets you. We are biologically wired for connection. It lowers cortisol, improves immune function, and yeah, probably helps more than your mushroom coffee/hot cocoa.

Build Your Biostack Instead

Feeling fine isn't the same as being well. Most of us are functioning—but barely. We're caffeinated through the morning, wired at night, reactive to stress, and wondering why we don't feel like ourselves anymore. But because nothing is technically wrong, we convince ourselves this must just be adulting. Or parenting. Or hormones. Or us.

Here's the truth: your body is communicating with you all the time. Fatigue, cravings, brain fog, and mood swings—none of these are character flaws. They're signals. And ignoring them in favor of another hack only makes you feel more broken when it doesn't work. You're not broken. You've just been given tools that were never built for where you're starting.

When we shift to biostacking, we're not just building habits; we're building capacity. The capacity to bounce back after a rough night. The capacity to feel grounded in a stressful week. The capacity to trust your body instead of constantly managing or second-guessing it.

You don't need to chase wellness perfection. You just need a rhythm that supports your body, not drains it. That's what biostacking is. A rhythm. A scaffolding. A way to anchor your choices in what actually works for you.

8

Food Isn't the Enemy. It's Fuel

You've probably spent years trying to "get it right." Counting, tracking, measuring and avoiding carbs, fearing fat, and exhausting yourself to be good. Maybe you've followed plans that promised everything if you just stuck to the rules. Maybe you've blamed yourself when they didn't work. And somewhere along the way, food stopped being fuel—and started feeling like the enemy.

Let's flip that.

Here's the truth: your body is not trying to sabotage you. It's surviving. You want it to focus at work, play with your kids, lift heavy things, and survive your calendar. It needs fuel. Not just any fuel, quality fuel, ideally in reasonable ratios and times. Just like you wouldn't dump a handful of dirt into your gas tank and hope for the best, you can't feed your body whatever's convenient and expect it to perform.

So if you've been treating food like a moral test—*I was good today* or *I was so bad this weekend*—it's time to stop. Food isn't a grade. You're not in trouble. You don't need to earn or atone for eating. You just need a new framework for considering what you eat. A better filter.

One that helps you look at your plate and ask, "What is this doing for me?" Not in a punishment way. In a powerful way. When you learn to see food as fuel—not as a reward, a threat, or a willpower test—you start making choices that actually support your body.

The Build-a-Plate Blueprint

If food is fuel, then every time you eat, you're building something. A quick snack. A steady burn. A meal that holds you for hours. The key is knowing what to build and how.

So here's your blueprint:

Protein. Quality Fat. Fiber.

Every time. That's the trio. That's your food-as-fuel plate blueprint.

Let's break it down.

- **Protein** is your stay-full signal. It helps rebuild tissue, support your metabolism, and keep cravings in check. It's the long-haul driver of satisfaction.
- **Quality fat** helps your body absorb nutrients, eliminate toxins, regulate hormones, and feel satiated. (If you're constantly "still hungry," fat might be the missing piece.)
- **Fiber** is the unsung hero. It slows digestion, balances blood sugar, supports your gut, and keeps you full. Think of it as your internal traffic controller; it paces the whole system.

Most of us were taught to count calories or avoid certain foods. But that doesn't help us build a meal, it just trains us to fear it. This isn't about restriction. It's about structure. Because when you hit the trifecta—protein, fat, fiber—your body says, *Cool. I'm good. I can run on this.*

And this works whether you're eating eggs or oatmeal, takeout or tofu. It's not about what's "allowed;" it's about what balances your system so you're not crashing mid-morning or fighting hunger all afternoon.

Protein. Quality fat. Fiber.

Write it down. Put it on your fridge. (I have a magnet available for you.) Tattoo it on your brain. This is your new filter, not for perfection, but for function.

From Meal to Metabolism

We're so used to thinking in terms of calories or points or macros that we forget the whole point of food is to fuel the body. That's it; that's the job. Instead of asking, *Did this meet my macros? Was this low-carb enough?* Ask, *Will this hold me till 1:00? Will this keep me focused through my 3:00 p.m. meeting?*

Now we're thinking like a body that wants to function, not like a person stuck in food guilt. Here's how to calibrate (use these numbers as a baseline and experiment from here with what works best for you):

- **Snacks**: If you're grabbing something to bridge the gap between meals, you're looking for about two to three ounces of protein, plus some fat or fiber to slow the burn. That'll hold you for one to two hours.
- **Meals**: If you're sitting down to lunch or dinner, four to six ounces of protein (for female bodies) or six to eight ounces (for male bodies), plus your fiber and fat, will hold you for about four-ish hours.

This isn't about obsessing over numbers; it's about understanding how your body works. If your tank runs out halfway through your morning, you don't need more discipline. You need more protein. If you're hungry an hour later, it's not that you're broken; it's that your plate was underbuilt. This is where freedom starts, not in eating less, but in eating enough of what sustains you.

The Fiber-First Flip

Most people build their meals by starting with a protein: *I'm having chicken, now what goes with it?* Or, they start with the craving: *I want toast*, and then toast is the meal.

Here's the reframe: Start with the fiber. Build it backwards. Why? Because fiber, especially from vegetables and fruits, is the real anchor. It's the thing that slows down digestion, helps regulate blood sugar, keeps you full, feeds your gut, and makes the rest of your food work for you.

So play with this:

- Open the fridge and ask, *What veggies do I have?*
- Start with what's in season, what looks good, or what needs to be used
- Then add your protein and fat to support it.

This works whether you're making breakfast, throwing together a salad, or cobbling something out of random leftovers. It also works at restaurants, while traveling, with meal kits, and with picky eaters. It works because it's a principle, not a plan.

Start with fiber. Then add protein to hold you. Add fat to satisfy you. And let everything else fill in the blanks.

Your Plate's Order of Operations

It's not just what's on your plate; it's the order you eat it in. Enter food stacking, a fancy name for something incredibly simple.

The idea is that eating your fiber and protein first, followed by your starch or sugary foods, helps your body handle them better. Your blood sugar stays more stable. Your energy lasts longer. Your cravings don't come roaring back an hour later.

This isn't about micromanaging every bite; it's about using your biology to your advantage. Because here's what happens when we eat the chips or the bread first: We spike blood sugar → insulin floods the system → crash follows → hunger or fatigue hits → repeat.

But when you start with the stabilizers, fiber, and protein, that spike gets blunted. The carbs that follow don't hit your system like a freight train. Your body metabolizes them slowly, with way less drama.

So what does this look like in real life?

- **At a restaurant**: Start with the salad or the shrimp cocktail. Eat the bread after the appetizer, not while scanning the menu.
- **At home**: Grab the veggies and chicken first, then the rice. Or eat them together, but start with a few bites of the stabilizers.
- **At a party**: Go for the guac and veggie sticks before the chips. Yes, seriously.

You don't have to skip the fries. You just don't need them to be first in line.

Some people get rigid with this: "You must eat all your vegetables before touching anything else!" That's not how we roll. Think of it more like sequencing. Lead with the stabilizers. Let the starches follow.

It's a slight shift. And it changes how your body responds and how you feel afterward. That's the goal, right? Feel energized now and later.

Snack Like a Strategist, Not a Scavenger

Snacking is not a character flaw. Snacks are not a sign of weakness. They're just food scaled down. But here's where most people get tripped up: they treat snacks like a chance to graze, nibble, or quiet the hanger with whatever's nearby. And that's when the snack turns into a blood sugar rollercoaster that leaves you hungrier than before.

Let's fix that. The shift is to think about a snack as just a mini meal. The only difference between a meal and a snack is how much you're having at once, and therefore how long it's going to last you until you need to fuel again. Use the same tools, and scale them down.

That means it follows the same build-a-plate blueprint as your meals:

Protein. Quality fat. Fiber.

You might not hit all three every time, and that's okay. But the more of them you include, the longer the snack will hold you. Here's how to think about it:

- One macronutrient = a snack that lasts an hour. *(Example: just fruit, just nuts, just jerky)*
- Two macronutrients = almost 2 hours of energy. *(Example: apple + almonds. Greek yogurt + berries. Hummus + carrots)*
- All three = a mini-meal. 2 solid hours and walking into that next meal empowered to make quality choices *(Example: turkey roll-ups + veggies + a few olives)*

And this is where leftovers become your secret weapon. That piece of salmon from dinner? The extra roasted broccoli? A couple of forkfuls of yesterday's grain bowl? That's a snack.

A Way of Eating

I hope by now you can tell I don't do diets. This isn't about elimination, calorie counting, or obsessive tracking. It also isn't about eating hyperprocessed foods at timed intervals or squeezing all your nutrition into a few sacred hours. And it's absolutely not about forcing food choice dogma down anyone's throat.

This is a way of eating. A way that aligns with how the human body works. A way that supports, not stresses, your energy, your focus, your rhythms. A way that lets you show up for your life without having food dominate it.

To reiterate, here's what food as fuel looks like across the day:

- Eight to twelve servings of vegetables (yes, really)
- One to two servings of fruit
- Protein every time you eat
- Quality fat two to four times a day

Don't panic. This isn't about counting lettuce leaves. It's about checking in: *Did I get protein at breakfast? Have I had anything green today? What's missing from this plate that would help it hold me longer?*

If you build your plate with fiber, protein, and fat—again and again—your meals start working for you. You stop swinging between starvation and snack attacks. You no longer need to reset every Monday. You stop feeling like you're constantly "off track." And most importantly, you stop turning to follow every new fad diet and start listening to your body.

And once you learn what your body needs, you stop trying to "get it right" and start simply getting what works.

9

Hydrate Like It Matters

We've all heard it, "Drink more water." It's on every wellness checklist, every resolution list, every "get healthy" article. You'd think with all that awareness, most of us would be walking around as fully hydrated, radiant beams of energy.

Instead? We're tired. We're foggy. Our skin's dry. We're bloated or backed up. We feel—off. So what gives? We're drinking the water. We're carrying around the bottles and the Stanleys. We're aware.

Here's the thing we aren't taught: hydration isn't only about how much water you drink. It's about whether your body can use it. Drinking water and being hydrated are not the same thing. You can drink water all day long and still be dehydrated. Drinking water is about consumption. Hydration is about absorption. And your body doesn't absorb water efficiently unless the conditions are right—specifically, unless electrolytes (aka minerals) are present to help water move into your cells and stay there.

I saw this play out in real time during the summer of 2025. I was volunteering at a charity golf outing on one of those Northeast scorchers, over 100 degrees before the heat index. We were outside all day, and I must have gone through more bottles of water than I could count.

I was stationed at hole 15, right near the restrooms, and guess what? I didn't need them. Not once. Until I drank a bottle of water with my favorite electrolyte mix. Within minutes, I had to go.

Electrolytes, Explained

You've heard the word. You've seen it on neon sports drinks and probably absorbed the vague idea that electrolytes = hydration. But beyond that? It gets murky fast. So let's clear it up.

Electrolytes are just minerals that carry an electric charge. That's it. They're the reason your muscles contract, your heart beats, and your brain communicates with the rest of your body. The main players are sodium, potassium, calcium, magnesium, and chloride. If those sound familiar, it's because you're supposed to get them from real food and salt.

When people reach for electrolyte drinks, what they think they're getting is cellular hydration. What they often get? A sugar bomb in disguise.

Even the sugar-free versions? Still packed with chemicals to fake the taste, and those fake sugars can confuse your body's signals and microbiome just as much as the real thing. And some of these drinks will actually dehydrate you more. Because sugar, especially fake sugar, can act as an anti-nutrient, pulling minerals out of your body instead of replenishing them.

If you want to try an electrolyte mix? Cool. Just read the label. Look for products with no added sugar or weird coloring, and a short ingredient list you can pronounce. A quality source of salt and the addition of other minerals like potassium and magnesium. The goal is function, not flavor engineering.

And remember: you don't need "performance hydration" unless you're running a marathon or doing hot yoga for hours. You need functional hydration, the kind that keeps you sharp, calm, and steady in your day-to-day. Because let's be honest, hydration shouldn't require a marketing budget.

The Salt Scare

Now, I know what some of you are thinking: *But Jenn, isn't salt bad for us?* Here's the truth: Salt isn't the enemy—at least, not real salt.

But somewhere along the line, we got the message that salt = high blood pressure = bad. Full stop. And like so many things in wellness, the truth is way more nuanced—and a lot more helpful once you understand it.

Here's the deal: the white, refined table salt found in processed foods and fast food isn't the kind your body needs. It's been stripped of its natural mineral content, bleached, and filled with additives to prevent clumping. And yeah, that kind of salt, in the context of a processed-food-heavy life, can be a problem.

But real salt—like Celtic sea salt or dark pink Himalayan sea salt—is something else entirely. It's mineral-rich. It's unrefined. And it contains the full spectrum of trace minerals your body uses to balance fluids, support nerve function, and regulate blood pressure. Yes, you read that correctly: real salt can help stabilize blood pressure.

Because here's what most conventional medical training overlooks: there is a difference between salt and sodium. Salt, real salt, supports the relationship between sodium, potassium, calcium, and magnesium.

If you've been avoiding salt because you're "being good," you might actually be depriving your body of what it needs to stay regulated. And if you've been reaching for salty snacks when you're stressed or tired, there's a chance that's more than a craving. It might be your body trying to course-correct with what it's missing.

The bottom line is that you don't need to fear salt; you need to upgrade your salt. And once you do, don't be surprised if your energy, focus, sleep, and stress levels shift, too.

What Does Your Body Use Hydration For?

Ok, so now we understand that water + minerals = hydration. But what's happening in your body when you hydrate well? And what's going sideways when you don't?

Here's the short version: hydration is how your body runs. No big deal, right? Water (with minerals, and again, we'll get to that) is what makes nearly every system in your body function properly.

Here's a snapshot:

Brain + Mood

Your brain is around 75 percent water. When you're dehydrated, neurons don't fire efficiently, and even mild dehydration can mess with your focus, memory, and mood. That feeling where you can't concentrate and everything's just a little harder? That might not be stress; it might be a lack of proper hydration.

Nervous System + Electrical Signaling

Your body is electric. Literally. (Cue Marcia Griffiths and "The Electric Slide.") Your nervous system relies on minerals (called electrolytes) to transmit signals from your brain to every part of your body. When you're hydrated—with water and minerals—your system works like a steady Wi-Fi connection. When you're not? It's glitchy, slow, and sometimes fully offline.

Digestion + Elimination

Hydration powers peristalsis, the muscle contractions that move food and waste through your digestive tract. Without enough water, digestion slows down, waste sits longer, and bloating sets in. Think of water like the oil in your digestive engine—less friction, smoother function.

Warm water primarily supports this by stimulating the gut lining. That belly bloat you blame on food? Sometimes it's just stuck waste. Hydration keeps things moving.

Circulation + Blood Pressure

Water makes up a huge portion of your blood volume. When you're dehydrated, blood thickens, and the heart works harder to pump it. This can mess with blood pressure—either too low or too high—which is why quality salt helps stabilize blood pressure by supporting electrolyte balance.

Temperature Regulation

Sweating is how your body cools down. No hydration = no sweat = overheating. But also, in cold, dry air, you can still dehydrate; your body's just not signaling thirst the same way.

Cellular Function

Your cells need water to do anything: repair tissue, transport nutrients, and clear waste. But they don't just need water splashing around your bloodstream—they need water inside them. That's called cellular hydration, and it only happens when minerals are present to help pull water into the cell.

Symptoms We Don't Realize Are Dehydration

Let's play a game: how many of these symptoms have you blamed on something else?

- Afternoon brain fog
- Waking up tired, even after eight hours
- Random headaches
- Dry skin, sinus pressure, or sore throat

- Low energy that no coffee can fix
- Cravings you swear aren't emotional, even cravings for fruit (that's me, I get this one!)
- Mood swings, anxiety, or even that feeling of "off-ness" you can't name
- Trouble sleeping
- Dizziness or lightheadedness when you stand
- Muscle cramps or tension
- Feeling kind of sad for no reason

If you're nodding along, you're not alone. Now, all of these things could be caused by something else, and every single one of these can be linked to dehydration. Not the textbook *I feel thirsty* kind. The sneaky, cumulative kind that builds over time.

We tend to think dehydration only happens on a hot day or after a workout. Truthfully? Some of the biggest culprits are hiding in plain sight. And they're part of everyday life.

Let's start with the obvious villain: air conditioning. I know; I love AC, too. I've thanked it out loud in August. But here's the thing: Air conditioning doesn't just cool the air; it dries it. Which means it's drying you, too. If you've ever spent a day in a cold office or flown on a plane and felt inexplicably wiped out— congrats, you've experienced what I call stealth dehydration. You weren't sick. You were slowly being shriveled by recycled, conditioned air. It's the same in winter. Dry indoor heat, no sweating, and we forget to drink water. Add some wine with dinner, a latte in the morning, and boom—you're a raisin with Wi-Fi.

Now layer in the dietary stuff. Sugar? Major mineral robber. Same with caffeine. And don't get me wrong—I'm not saying never have your coffee. Most of my clients have two cups a day and love every sip. But if you're not replenishing what caffeine drains, you're running a deficit.

Processed foods and refined carbs act similarly. They dehydrate at the cellular level, offering nothing in return.

Then there are the things we think are helping—like Gatorade. I already mentioned the impact of any brightly colored "electrolyte" drink packed with sugar, artificial colors, and a side of guilt. These drinks are marketed as recovery aids, but they're often just fancy sugar water. More sugar = more mineral loss. It's like bailing out a leaky boat with a colander.

And finally, there's soda—Coke, Pepsi, all of it. Aside from the sugar, many contain phosphoric acid, which can pull calcium out of your bones. I'm not being dramatic. You can clean a car engine with cola. Think about that the next time your brain says, *I'm thirsty*, and you reach for a can. But I digress…

These things aren't just "not hydrating." They're actively undoing the hydration your body's trying to hold onto.

What Real Rehydration Looks Like

At this point, we've untangled the biggest hydration myths. You know drinking water alone isn't enough. You know minerals matter. And you know that Gatorade isn't your hero. So the question becomes—what is?

Let's start here: Rehydration isn't a detox plan, a gallon-a-day challenge, or a performance supplement regimen. It's about supporting your body so it can use what you give it. And the good news? It's way simpler than we've been led to believe.

Here's what works:

1. **Salt your water, on purpose.**
Add a pinch of Celtic sea salt to your water bottle. That's it. Not a scoop, not a tablespoon. Just enough to make the water taste pleasantly different—not salty, not flat. Your body knows what it needs. When the water tastes enjoyable to you, you've likely hit the sweet spot (salty spot?). It's a simple, low-cost way to support actual absorption instead of just chasing volume.

2. **Consider Cal-Mag.**
Calcium and magnesium are both critical for hydration, especially when it comes to your nervous system. They help regulate

muscle function, relaxation, sleep, and mood. If you're feeling wired but tired, tense, or irritable, it could be more than stress—it might be a mineral deficiency. A quality Cal-Mag supplement can support your system in a way plain water never could. Look for one that's pH balanced and bioavailable, not the chalky kind from the drugstore aisle.

3. Eat your minerals.

You don't have to supplement everything (in fact, please don't). You can eat your way to better hydration, too. Some of the best whole food sources of electrolytes include:

- Leafy greens (magnesium, potassium, calcium)
- Avocados (potassium, magnesium)
- Sweet potatoes (potassium)
- Nuts and seeds (magnesium, calcium)
- Seaweed (sodium and trace minerals)

These foods aren't just healthy in the vague wellness-speak way. They're delivering the minerals your cells need to pull in and hold onto water.

4. Pay attention to your inputs and outputs.

If you're drinking water and still feeling off, ask:

- Are you replenishing minerals or just flushing them?
- Are you drinking soda, coffee, or alcohol that pulls hydration out?
- Are you getting dizzy, moody, bloated, or foggy in the afternoons?

These are signs your system might be off-balance.

How Much Is Enough? And Can You Have Too Much?

Once people understand that hydration is more than just drinking water, the next question is always: So, how much should I drink? The short answer: more than you think, and less than you fear.

There are a few common guidelines floating around:

- The classic "8 by 8" rule: eight 8-ounce glasses, or 64 ounces a day
- Half your body weight in ounces
- The CDC guideline: about 2.7 liters per day (roughly 90 to 95 ounces for women)

And here's the truth? Any of those can work. What matters is that you choose one and use it as a target, not a judgment. Notice your current baseline, pay attention to how you feel, and move in the direction of one of these guidelines.

Some days you'll need more. Hot weather, a workout, more caffeine or alcohol, dry indoor air, all of these raise your hydration needs. Other days, you might hit your goal without even thinking about it.

The important part is consistency. Your body loves rhythm. The more regularly you hydrate, the less work your system has to do to recalibrate.

Now, what about too much? It's rare, but yes, you can overdo it. Drinking excessive amounts of water in a short time (think five or six liters at once) can dilute your blood's sodium levels and cause a dangerous condition called hyponatremia. This mostly happens to athletes who over-hydrate during endurance events without replenishing electrolytes.

For most people, overhydration isn't the risk. Under-absorption is. If you're constantly drinking, constantly peeing, and still thirsty or foggy—that's not too much water; that's water without minerals. Occasionally, constant thirst is a sign of something else happening in the body. If you're paying attention to hydration, absorption, and minerals and still find yourself constantly thirsty, be sure to consult your healthcare provider.

Everyday Hydration Habits That Stick

Once you understand what hydration is, the next step is building habits that make it sustainable.

Here are some real-world ways to make hydration easier to maintain:

1. **Keep it visible.**

Out of sight, out of sip. If your water is tucked in a bag or buried under your desk, you'll forget. Keep a large bottle out in the open: on your desk, your nightstand, your kitchen counter.

2. **Set gentle cues.**

You don't need an app or hourly alarm (unless you want one). Simply find natural anchors: after you brush your teeth, when you're preparing each meal, when you sit down at your computer, right before you grab your coffee. Tie your hydration to routines you already do.

3. **Choose a container you'll actually use.**

A bottle with a straw, a glass you love, a tumbler that fits your car cupholder. If it's easy to carry, easy to open, and feels good in your hand, you'll drink more. Function leads to follow-through.

4. **Use temperature to your advantage.**

Some people find cold water refreshing. Others can only drink it if it's room temp or warm. Hot water can support digestion, especially first thing in the morning and with fresh lemon juice. Bottom line: Drink the water you'll actually drink. That's the right temperature.

5. Add flavor—naturally.

If plain water feels boring, dress it up. Add lemon, lime, orange slices, cucumber, mint, or a pinch of sea salt. You can make it taste better and work better for your body. Skip the sugary flavor packets and artificial drops. Pro Tip 1: The longer the fruit, veggie, or herb is submerged in water, the stronger its flavor will be. Pro Tip 2: Combine the flavors. Not only does it make you feel a bit fancy or reminiscent of a spa, but the flavors are that much better, and it can cut the bitterness that can come from the rind. Go for cucumber and mint, lemon and lime, grapefruit and orange slices. Try it, I think you'll like it.

6. Aim slightly higher than you need.

Research shows that when people aim for a specific target, they often fall a bit short. So give yourself a buffer. If your target is 80 ounces, aim for 100. If you need three bottles a day, fill four. Overshooting your goal helps you actually hit it. And, as we're re-learning with each chapter, know thyself. If having a few ounces left at the end of the day is going to make you beat yourself up or feel like a failure, skip this idea! You do you. That is absolutely the best approach.

10

Move Your Mass

I t's one of the few things most experts agree on: exercise is good for us. Great, even. Vital for heart health, mood, bone density, blood sugar, stress management—you name it.

And yet, a lot of us feel weirdly bad about it. Like we're always behind, always doing it wrong, or just—not doing enough. The pressure is relentless: more steps, more sweat, more toning, more burn, and more soreness.

For something we're told to do daily, movement comes with a surprising amount of guilt, confusion, and straight-up misinformation. We've been handed workout plans that don't match our bodies, chased results that never materialized, and internalized a lot of judgment about how fitness should look.

Let's uncomplicate it. This chapter is not about giving you one more routine to follow. It's about cutting through the noise to clarify what truly supports your metabolism, your hormones, and your long-term strength, especially as you age. It's about helping you understand the difference between what burns calories and what builds a body that burns fuel more effectively.

It's about swapping the obsession with exercise to undo our food choices for a real relationship with movement that is rooted in function, flexibility, and the kind of strength that makes your life easier.

Your body was built to move. And when you move your mass—whether that means lifting heavy, walking daily, stretching gently, or sprinting with intention—you're signaling to your body that it matters.

Your body was built to move. And when you do, even in small, imperfect ways, you're sending powerful biochemical signals that say, *I want to feel confident in this body, and I'm showing up for it.*

Let's Right-Size Our Cardio

For decades, we were told that cardio was the key to weight loss and metabolism. Just move more, burn more, and the scale will follow. As we've started to understand the body more holistically—and especially as women move through their 30s, 40s, and beyond—it's become clear that cardio doesn't offer all the benefits our bodies and our minds crave.

Now, let's not throw cardio under the bus. It supports heart health and brain function, and can also be a fantastic mood booster. Yet when it becomes your go-to strategy for fat loss or metabolism, especially as your hormones shift, your go-to cardio regimen often backfires. Long, steady-state cardio—think an hour on the treadmill or zoning out in spin class—raises cortisol, your body's primary stress hormone. That's natural and expected during exercise, but when life is already a cortisol cocktail of deadlines, family logistics, poor sleep, and blood sugar swings, and then you throw in more stress via endless cardio? Your system stays stuck in red alert, and instead of burning fat, your body holds onto it as a protective mechanism. (Hey, it takes a lot of stored energy to run from a saber-toothed tiger 24/7.)

This is why short bursts of intensity followed by recovery, like interval training, tend to be more effective for fat removal and metabolic support. Think 20 to 30 minutes, not an hour. Think jog-walk-jog-walk, or lunges/squats-abs-lunges/squats-abs, not jog-forever-and-hope.

Why? Because intervals give you the hormonal benefits without the chronic stress load. They raise your heart rate, fire up your body's engines, and then let your system exhale, literally and figuratively.

And before you panic: no, this doesn't mean you have to do burpees until you see stars. "Intensity" is relative. For one person, that's a hill sprint. For someone else, it's power walking up a staircase.

And if you're someone who loves long cardio—the rhythm, the alone time, the mental reset—fantastic!. Keep your soulmate workouts. Build a routine that includes them without making them the center of your fitness strategy or everyday movement. Prolonged or intense cardio can be your bonus, not your baseline.

You get to love movement and be strategic about it.

At the end of the day, your workouts must work for your body, not against your hormones or health goals.

Muscle is the New Metabolism

Okay, so if cardio isn't the secret to lasting fat removal or a faster metabolism, what is? That would be muscle.

Muscle isn't just for athletes or fitness influencers. It's not about looking a certain way or chasing some kind of shredded Instagram body. Muscle is about function. It's about strength, stability, and metabolic health. And most of all, it's about what keeps you well as you age.

Starting in your late 20s, you naturally begin to lose muscle mass—around one to two percent per year if you're not actively maintaining it. By your 40s, that adds up quickly. This process, known as sarcopenia, doesn't just show up as feeling a little weaker. It affects your balance, mobility, metabolism, and even blood sugar regulation. It accelerates aging as our bodies begin to move and process energy differently.

Muscle plays a huge role in your resting metabolic rate, which is the number of calories your body burns just keeping you alive. The more lean muscle you have, the more energy your body requires to maintain it, even when you're just sitting on the couch or sleeping. That's why people with more muscle often feel like their metabolism is faster.

Beyond the metabolic math, muscle gives you more freedom in your life. It's what helps you get up off the floor without needing three pieces of furniture. It's what lets you carry your groceries in one trip, pick up your kids or grandkids, move through your day without pain, and get up off the toilet by yourself when you're over 80. It's what keeps your body resilient when the unexpected happens.

Now, let's also address the elephant in the room. When I talk about building muscle, many women immediately worry about "getting bulky." Let me be clear: that is not a concern for the vast majority of people. Building visible, bulky muscle takes massive effort (specific training, a surplus of food), and often higher levels of testosterone than most women naturally have. You are far more likely to develop the lean, strong, toned look that so many women are after by lifting heavy enough to truly challenge your muscles.

Call it "muscle mass," call it "toning," call it "long, lean lines" if that's more comfortable for you. Whatever you call it, the point is the same: your body needs it. Muscle protects you. It stabilizes you. It powers you through life.

And no, this doesn't mean you need to live at the gym. It means working with resistance—safely, consistently, and with enough effort to matter—two to four times per week. It means challenging your muscles to do something hard, so they have a reason to adapt and grow. It can be bodyweight. It can be dumbbells. It can be resistance bands. The tool is less important than the intent.

If you've been chasing fat removal through cardio alone and not seeing results, this is your invitation to shift focus.

This isn't about getting ripped. It's about staying capable—in your 40s, 70s, and beyond, and everywhere in between. Muscle gives you options. It gives you power. And it's never too late to start building more of it.

How to Strength Train Effectively (With or Without Equipment)

So, we know muscle is essential for your metabolism, your strength, and your long-term health. But how do you build it? By challenging your muscles.

Strength training is about asking your muscles to do something hard enough that they have a reason to grow. That doesn't require equipment. Resistance is resistance. Your muscles don't care whether the load comes from a dumbbell, a resistance band, your own bodyweight, or gravity. They just know they're being asked to show up.

Bodyweight workouts can be incredibly effective—if you're pushing yourself. That might mean slowing down a movement, holding tension at the bottom of a squat, or adjusting the angle of a pushup. The goal is effort. Form. Focus. Not fancy tools. Many people would build strength faster doing bodyweight movements with intention than flinging around weights with zero strategy.

Of course, adding resistance helps. Bands, dumbbells, and even a backpack full of books can increase the challenge. I did this in college. I'd put a bunch of textbooks in a backpack and walk. I was ahead of my time. Today's internet would call it a weighted vest or rucking. If access or budget is a barrier, I'm calling BS (sorry, not sorry); that's not a reason to tap out. You already have the most important tool: your body. What matters is how you use it.

And one more thing, don't get stuck thinking it has to take an hour. Five focused minutes count. A fifteen-minute circuit on your lunch break counts. A single challenging set between Zoom calls? That counts too.

Whether you're lifting a barbell or your own body, the principle is the same: if it's hard, it's working. Challenge, not equipment, drives results.

No, You Can't Spot Train

Let's rip off this Band-Aid quickly: You cannot spot reduce fat. You just can't.

You can do all the crunches in the world and still have belly fat. You can plank until your shoulders cry, tricep dip until bed, and still feel like something is hanging under your arms. That doesn't mean you're doing it wrong. It means your body is doing exactly what it's designed to do.

Because here's the truth: fat removal happens systemically, not locally. Meaning, your metabolism works body-wide. Not in zones. Not in little pin-pointed fat pockets that melt away just because you decided to do extra squats this week. You can build muscle in a specific area. That's why we have "leg day" and "arm day," along with targeted movements.

But building muscle ≠ removing fat in that exact location. Let's say that again, louder for the people in the back: Muscle growth and fat removal are two different processes. Removing fat depends on your hormones, stress levels, sleep, nutrition, and overall movement patterns, not the number of lunges you do.

And there's another layer here: Your body decides where it stores fat and where it lets it go. That's not willpower. That's genetics and hormones. For women, that often means belly, hips, thighs, and arms. And especially as we move through perimenopause and menopause, the hormonal shifts can change where fat wants to hang out.

This is where so many people get frustrated because they think they're failing. When really, they're just up against a giant myth. So let's shift the goal.

Instead of chasing "arm fat" or "muffin tops" or "lower belly pooch," focus on:

- Building muscle across your body
- Supporting your metabolism with food, sleep, and stress management
- Moving consistently in ways your body enjoys and can recover from

Because this is the kind of holistic approach that yields results.

How to Know You're Doing Enough

One of the most common questions I hear, whether it's from longtime podcast listeners, clients, or someone just getting started, is, "How do I know if I'm doing enough?"

And underneath that question is usually a swirl of doubt. *Am I lifting heavy enough? Should I be sore? Should I be doing more days, more reps, more minutes? Should I already be seeing results?*

First, take a breath. That feeling of uncertainty doesn't mean you're doing it wrong. It means you care. You're paying attention. And that's a powerful thing.

Now let's get into it.

You're probably doing enough if...

- The last few reps of your set feel genuinely hard, but not sloppy
- Your muscles feel challenged and a little fatigued after a workout, even if you're not wrecked
- You're gradually getting stronger or more stable: lifting a little more, holding a plank a little longer, recovering faster

- You're not constantly sore, and if/when you are, it fades within a couple of days and doesn't interfere with daily life

You might need to level up if...

- You're breezing through workouts without breaking a sweat or losing form
- You've been lifting the same weights for months, and it's not challenging anymore
- You feel like you're doing "all the things" but seeing zero change in energy, strength, or body composition
- You're bored. (Yes, that counts. Bored muscles are muscles that aren't being asked to adapt.)

And let's clear something up while we're here: Soreness is not a measure of success. I know, this one hits me hard too. I crave that feeling sometimes. Yes, it can be a sign you've worked new muscle fibers or pushed your usual edge. But if you're limping for three days after every session, that's not a badge of honor; that's a recovery problem. And if you're never sore at all, but you're progressing in strength and stability? That's a win. Don't chase pain; chase progress.

Also, fatigue is normal. But form breakdown is a signal. If you're doing squats and suddenly your knees are caving in, or your back is arching during a press, it's time to stop or scale back. More isn't better. Better is better.

Here's a helpful reframe:

Doing "enough" isn't about maxing out every session. It's about asking enough of your body that it has a reason to adapt and then giving it the support to do so. That means challenge, yes. But also food. Sleep. Rest. Movement that feels like effort, yet doesn't hijack your whole day or leave you crawling out of the gym.

When in doubt, track your energy, not just your metrics. Do you feel more capable? Are stairs easier? Is your posture better?

Are you more present in your body and less at war with it? If the answer's yes, even in small ways, you're doing enough.

Rest ≠ Weakness

There's a toxic little idea that's still floating around in too many fitness spaces: that rest is for the undisciplined. Let's put that to bed right now. Rest isn't quitting; rest is strategy. It's not what happens when you "fall off track;" it's part of the track.

Every time you strength train, you're creating tiny microtears in your muscle fibers. That soreness you feel the next day? That's your body healing. And it's through that healing process that the muscle gets stronger.

If you're skipping rest because you're "being good" or "staying on top of it," you're just getting in your own way. Recovery isn't optional.

That doesn't mean you need to lie on the couch for forty-eight hours bingeing true crime documentaries (though no judgment if you do—been there!). Recovery can be active, meaning walking, stretching, foam rolling, or doing something gentle and restorative. It's about giving the systems you've stressed time to recalibrate.

And this is where a little nuance is helpful. If your workouts are high-intensity—think heavy lifting or intervals—you'll likely need more recovery between sessions. If your movement is lower impact or moderate, like walking or mobility work, you can do that daily without burning out your system (provided we're supporting with nutrition, hydration, sleep, etc.).

A helpful rule of thumb? Take at least one full rest day each week. And maybe don't go more than two days in a row without moving your body in some way. Movement begets movement. The more consistently you stay in rhythm, the easier it is to keep going.

Now, if you're the type who struggles to take a day off—if skipping a workout makes you feel anxious or behind—that's a flag, too. Discipline is a great tool, until it turns into rigidity.

Listen, I'm type A too. I love a plan. *And* health is bigger than any calendar. The goal is sustainability, not streaks. Longevity, not burnout.

If your body's asking for rest, give it. If your schedule throws off your routine, adapt. If the chaos of life has you sleeping four hours a night and eating cookies for breakfast, maybe your best move isn't another bootcamp class; it's a walk and a nap. Rest isn't weakness. It's wisdom. And honoring that doesn't make you less committed. It makes you someone who understands how human bodies work.

Stretching Isn't Optional

If strength training is the foundation, and cardio is the support beam, then flexibility is the part we tend to ignore until something creaks, snaps, or screams. Stretching isn't just a warm-up or cool-down. It's not an extra. It's not a "bonus if you have time." It's a core part of keeping your body functional, injury-resistant, and responsive as you age. And yet, so many of us skip it.

We treat stretching like flossing. Not doing it means we can reclaim a couple of minutes in the day. And we know we should do it, but unless there's pain, we don't make it a priority. Until suddenly, there's pain.

Here's why it matters: a flexible muscle is a functional muscle. When you strength train, you contract muscle fibers. When you stretch, you elongate them. You're giving your muscles space to recover, recalibrate, and keep doing their job without pulling on your joints like an overworked rubber band.

Tight muscles don't just limit range of motion; they mess with your alignment. That's where you get compensations, strain, and eventually injury. Ever tweak your lower back doing something simple, like bending over to tie your shoes? That's not bad luck. That's usually tight hamstrings, hips, or both.

As we age, our muscles naturally get tighter. It's part of the body's way of protecting the joints, especially when hormones shift and recovery slows. But tightness isn't inevitable. And it's not permanent.

Let's talk types:

Static stretching is what most people know: holding a position and breathing through it. Useful, especially post-workout.

Dynamic stretching is more movement-based. Think leg swings, walking lunges, or jumping jacks. Great as a warm-up because it preps your nervous system without shocking cold muscles.

And then there's mobility, a more integrated approach that focuses not just on lengthening muscles, but on improving how your joints move and how your body moves as a whole. You don't need to be a yogi or be able to drop into the splits. You do need to be able to twist, bend, reach, and get up off the floor without making it an Olympic event.

Stretching daily, even for just five to ten minutes, can make a noticeable difference in how you feel, recover, and perform. Think of it like brushing your teeth for your muscles. It keeps things clean, smooth, and working the way they're supposed to. And as a bonus? Stretching helps with soreness, sleep, stress, and even digestion. No protein powder on the planet can offer all of that.

So yes, strength matters. And flexibility is what allows that strength to show up in your life. Don't skip it. Don't save it for later. Build it in, now.

Bring in Balance

There's one more piece of the movement puzzle that doesn't get nearly enough airtime, especially in mainstream fitness, and that's balance. As I continue to coach, learn, and evolve, I've started talking about movement in four core elements: cardio, strength, flexibility, and balance. Not that the fitness industry is quite there yet, but we're always a few steps ahead over here.

Balance isn't just about standing still on one foot or mastering yoga poses. It's about training your body to stabilize under pressure quickly, automatically, and without you having to think about it. And just like strength or flexibility, it's a skill you can build.

The good news? It doesn't require a whole separate routine. You can weave balance work into what you're already doing. Try standing on one foot while brushing your teeth or brewing your coffee. Want more? Do your bicep curls or shoulder presses on one leg. Shift your weight while you wash dishes. Play with arm positions, such as hands in a T, in prayer, or overhead. Just make sure you're not locking the knee joint or sinking into the hip of your standing leg. (Yes, I see you.)

Balance tends to be one of those investments that pays off way down the road. Maybe you catch yourself when stepping over a puddle next week. The bigger payoff, though, comes decades from now, when your reflexes kick in to prevent a fall that could've broken a hip. Most fractures in our later years start with a loss of balance. This is prevention at its most powerful.

So yes, we can talk about wanting balance in our nutrition and our lives. But also—literally, physically—balance. It's what keeps us upright, agile, and independent. And it's worth practicing now.

Shoes, Sweat, and Shiny Objects

The fitness world has never met a gimmick it didn't love. Ankle weights, EMS belts, detox wraps, vibrating platforms, vibrating belts, pre-workout powders promising superhuman strength—if it's shiny and promises faster results, someone's probably trying to sell it to you.

Let's simplify. First: You don't need gear to get fit. You don't need a $300 wearable, a $200 pair of leggings, or a Bluetooth-connected foam roller to build strength. Tools can be helpful. Yet your body is already equipped with everything you need to get started.

Let's break a few things down:

Ankle and wrist weights.

They might sound like an excellent idea for leveling up your walk or everyday movements, but in most cases, they're not doing much beyond adding strain to your joints, especially your knees, hips, and shoulders. If you're recovering from an injury or working with a physical therapist or professional to help with form, sure. Otherwise? Skip them and focus on intentional resistance training instead.

Pre-workout drinks.

Some can be helpful, especially if they include quality protein or branched-chain amino acids, maybe some quality carbohydrates, and you haven't eaten. But many are just caffeine bombs in neon-colored packaging. If the ingredient list reads like a chemistry final, it's probably not fueling your body in a meaningful way. Real food, real hydration, and consistent movement will always do more than a scoop of mystery powder.

Electric stimulation (like Emsculpt).

There's some emerging research here, and some people do feel results. But let's be honest: nothing replaces the benefits of voluntary movement. You can stimulate a muscle all day, but if there's a layer of fat over it—or if your nutrition, sleep, and stress are out of whack—you're not going to see long-term change. And the price tag? You could buy a year's worth of groceries that support your goals instead.

Shoes and gear.

This one's personal. Some people feel better lifting barefoot or in flat shoes. Others need arch support or feel stronger in sneakers. What matters is that your gear supports your movement, not that it fits a trend. Pay attention to how your body feels, not how your workout looks on Instagram.

And finally, celebrity trainer routines, fitfluencer challenges, or one-size-fits-all workout calendars might look impressive, but they aren't necessarily built for your body, your goals, your hormones, or your schedule. What works for someone else's red carpet prep probably won't translate to your Tuesday morning.

Here's the real flex—discernment. Knowing what's worth your effort and what's just noise.

The truth is, most of the shiny stuff promises shortcuts. Wellness isn't a hack; it's a habit. And the more you focus on simple, sustainable actions (lifting heavy, walking more, sleeping well, fueling smart), the less you'll feel tempted by the hype.

No gadget can replace consistency. No supplement can replace sleep. No shortcut can replace showing up for yourself. Before you buy, swallow, or strap anything on, ask yourself, *What problem is this solving, and do I actually need it solved?* Chances are, your body already knows the answer.

Even When Life Gets Messy

Let's be honest, there's a difference between what we know to do and what happens when real life shows up.

You can have the perfect workout plan, a brand-new set of weights, and the best intentions. Then comes a sick kid, a work deadline, a travel week, a string of restless nights, or a stretch of days when you're just not feeling it. And in those moments, it's easy to think you blew it.

Here's the reframe: consistency doesn't mean repetition. It doesn't mean showing up exactly the same way every day. That's not real life. That's a Xerox copy. (Remember those? Hello, 1990s.)

Consistency means you keep going, even if it looks different. Even if your workout today is five squats, a few stretches, and a walk to the mailbox. Even if you're not "in the mood."

Even if you're navigating the messiest season you've had in years. Movement doesn't need to be perfect to be powerful.

Some weeks, twenty minutes a day might feel luxurious. Other weeks, you might be stacking movement into tiny moments, such as ten pushups before your shower, a plank hold while your coffee brews, a quick walk after lunch. That all counts. Every minute counts.

And not just for your muscles, but for your mind. Movement shifts your chemistry. It helps metabolize stress, steady your blood sugar, and reconnect you to your body, especially when everything else feels chaotic. If you're traveling, move differently. If you're busy, get creative. If you're tired, make it gentler. Don't talk yourself out of it just because it doesn't look like it "should."

Because you're not just moving your body. You're reinforcing your identity. You're someone who moves. Someone who takes care of themselves. Someone who understands that strength isn't built despite life; it's built inside of it.

On the days when it all feels like too much, remember this: You don't need the perfect conditions. You don't need the perfect energy. You just need to move your mass. That's it. That's enough. That's the win.

11

Not to Be Dramatic, But Stress Is Killing You

I hate to say it like this because it sounds dramatic, but it's true: The stress response that was designed to keep us alive is also what's slowly breaking us down.

Back in the day—like caveman, saber-tooth tiger kind of back—the stress response was a life-saving gift. You see a bear. Your brain lights up. Cortisol floods your system, your muscles get a surge of energy, and nonessential functions shut down so you can run like hell. That's the fight-or-flight response in action. And thank goodness for it.

Here's the problem: The modern version of "the bear" never leaves the room. We're not running from predators anymore;

we're just drowning in Slack notifications, over-scheduled pre-teens, looming deadlines, and the nagging voice in our head that won't quit. Our bodies don't know the difference between a lion attack and an overflowing inbox. They just react. What was meant to be a short-term, emergency response has become our all-the-time operating system.

That stress response—cortisol up, everything else down—used to save our lives. Now? It's quietly sabotaging our reproduction, metabolism, immune system, mental clarity, and weight. And because stress isn't something we can see or measure easily, most of us don't realize it's what's driving our cravings, our fatigue, our belly fat, our infertility, and our *Why can't I get it together?* spiral.

You're not weak. You're not broken. You're living in a body that was built for one kind of danger in a world that gives you a different kind every five minutes. This chapter is about helping you see this clearly so you can start changing your relationship with it. Because the problem isn't that we have stress. The problem is that we don't know how to complete it.

Modern Life Is a Stress Loop

Working from your couch in leggings shouldn't feel like a survival sport—but it does to your body. Here's what's wild: Most of us don't think of ourselves as stressed out. Not in a crisis-mode, white-knuckle kind of way. But if I asked you how often you feel calm, actually peaceful, what would you say? Exactly.

The truth is, we're all living in a kind of low-key emergency mode because the way modern life is structured leaves no real off-switch. Work lives in our pockets. Parenting is 24/7. Even "self-care" can feel like another task we're failing at. And don't get me started on the news cycle because even when you just want to stay informed, it's a steady drip of cortisol.

Stress has become ambient. That's especially true if you're working from home. Maybe you've lost track of what day it is (because every day is kind of—all the days). Maybe your kitchen table is your desk (mine is), your kids' classroom, and where you collapse with a glass of wine at night. There's no boundary anymore between "on" and "off." So we just stay "on," burning through energy reserves we never get a chance to replenish.

Even the things we used to rely on to help us de-stress—like gym classes, friend dates, or that happy hour that made Thursdays feel like Fridays—might be harder to access now. Although we've "recovered" from COVID, many of us continue to work from home and struggle to make time for things that used to be nonnegotiable. And that's not nothing. Because those outlets weren't just "nice to have." They were the things that helped us complete the stress cycle.

So what happens when all the input stays high, and all the output disappears? We get stuck. Stuck in a loop of low-grade overwhelm that spikes cravings, tanks our mood, disrupts our sleep, and leaves us wondering why we can't just "handle it better." And the worst part? We blame ourselves. We think, *Other people seem to be coping; why am I so tired all the time?*

But you're not failing. You're not lazy. You're living in a system that never shuts off, and your body is doing its best to keep up.

Stress Is Chemistry, Not Character

Let's clear something up. Your inability to "just relax," your craving for chocolate at 9:00 p.m., the procrastination that seems like it's becoming your personality, and the fact that you haven't done that workout you bookmarked last week—none of that is a personal failure. It's chemistry.

When we talk about stress, we tend to focus on how it feels—anxious, overwhelmed, irritable, and wired but tired. What's happening is biochemical. Your brain detects a threat—real or perceived—and *boom*. Cortisol floods your system. That hormone isn't bad; it's also what gets us out of bed in the morning.

But cortisol doesn't work alone. When it spikes, it suppresses other systems so your body can prioritize survival. That means your immune system goes quiet. Your digestion slows. Your metabolism taps the brakes. Your reproductive system sends out-of-office signals. Even your higher-level brain functions, such as decision-making and impulse control, are dialed down.

Why? Because in a crisis, your body doesn't care if you can spell "quinoa." It just wants to keep you alive. This is why stress messes with your health in ways that don't feel related. It's why you catch colds more easily. Why you gain weight without changing your eating habits. Why you forget what you walked into the room for. And it's also why you reach for sugar.

Cortisol makes your body crave quick energy—fast carbs, caffeine, comfort food—because that's what you'd need to out-run a bear. The chemical cascade is real. These cravings are not about discipline. They're about your biology doing its job.

So let's just take willpower off the table for a second. You're not weak. You're not "addicted to sugar." You're a person with stress hormones doing precisely what they were designed to do.

The problem is that in today's world, the stressors don't go away. You're not running from the bear, collapsing safely in a cave, and letting your cortisol come back down. You're just getting a new email, seeing a new headline, answering another question from your kid, hearing your phone buzz, remembering that you forgot to order groceries. Again. And so the cortisol stays up. And up. And up.

When that happens, your metabolism slows. Your body holds on to fat, especially around your midsection, as a way to store energy for the next emergency. Your blood sugar rises because your body thinks you'll need it readily available to fuel your muscles. And over time, that high blood sugar can make your cells stop responding to insulin efficiently. That's how chronic stress contributes to insulin resistance, and eventually, conditions like diabetes.

Let that sink in: it's not just that stress makes you feel lousy. It's that it changes how your body functions. So no, this isn't in your head. And no, it's not something you can just "push through." This is the part completely ignored by the adage, "Just eat clean and work out." Because none of that works if your body is living in survival mode.

We don't fix stress with hacks or hustle. We fix it by respecting the chemistry and learning how to shift it.

What Happens If We Don't Interrupt It?

We like to think stress is temporary. A bad day. A tough week. Something you can shake off with a glass of wine and a night of sleep. But the body doesn't keep stress on a calendar.

If we don't complete the cycle—if we don't give our body the signals that the threat has passed—then stress doesn't leave. It just settles in. And when it settles in, it starts to reshape everything.

Chronically elevated cortisol doesn't just cause cravings or fatigue. It changes how your body stores fat. It messes with your ability to build muscle. It slows your thyroid, disrupts your sex hormones, and puts the brakes on your metabolism. And it doesn't do this in some abstract "stress is bad for you" kind of way. It does it mechanistically, like flipping off switches inside your system.

Your body is trying to protect you. But when the "danger" never ends, the protection becomes a problem. Eventually, that system can burn out.

This is what we call adrenal fatigue—when the stress response has been stuck in overdrive for so long that the system just gives up. Cortisol drops too low, not because you're relaxed, but because your adrenal glands are tapped out. You still feel anxious and wired, but now you're also exhausted at 6:00 p.m., then wide awake around 11:00 p.m.. Your sleep is worse. Your recovery tanks. Your body is confused. You're confused.

And of course, it's all invisible. There's no headline for this. No emergency-room moment. Just the slow slide of not feeling like yourself. Of thinking, *Why am I so tired? Why can't I lose weight? Why does everything feel harder than it used to?* You might even convince yourself it's just part of getting older. It's not. It's chronic stress, unprocessed.

Here's the thing: you're not meant to live in this state. Survival mode was designed to be short-term. When it becomes your normal, it doesn't just wear you down; it shuts you down.

So if any of this sounds familiar—if your brain is foggy, your cravings are loud, and your motivation is gone—please hear me. You're not lazy. You're not doing it wrong. You're just overdue for a reset.

Okay, So What Actually Helps?

Here's the truth: stress isn't going anywhere. Inbox zero isn't real. Kids don't suddenly become self-sufficient. The news isn't about to become calming.

Good news! Your body doesn't need the stress to disappear; it just needs to know the emergency is over. This is the piece of the puzzle too often glossed over: stress is a cycle. And that cycle needs to be completed. Not with another green juice or productivity hack, but with simple, science-backed ways to tell your body, *we're safe now.*

Let's talk about them.

Laugh. (No, seriously.)
Laughter triggers the release of endorphins and lowers cortisol. And no, it doesn't have to be deep or poetic. Scroll Instagram memes. Watch that dumb video your friend texted. Even a forced smile—yes, literally faking it—can create a chemical shift. One of my favorite experts talks about holding a smile for ten seconds. That facial expression alone can start to drop cortisol and boost your feel-good hormones. It's not about pretending things are fine. It's about reminding your body that you're not in danger.

Breathe like you mean it.
When you're stressed, your breath becomes shallow and high up in your chest—like that involuntary gasp when someone startles you. It's a signal to your nervous system that you're under threat.

To flip that signal, breathe from your diaphragm. Place your hands on your ribcage and feel your ribs expand like an accordion. Use this rhythm: Inhale for six seconds, hold for four, and exhale for eight. Breathe through your nose, and let the exhale drag across your vocal cords so it makes a sound. That sound plus the counting activates both sides of your brain, which means you literally *can't* think about anything else while you're doing it. It brings you into the present and gives your stress response a full-body exhale.

Community builds immunity.

Isolation fuels the stress cycle. Connection interrupts it. Even virtual connection helps—Zoom happy hours, calling a friend to vent or discuss the latest celeb tea, group texts full of silly jokes, sharing memes like it's your job (I know it's not just me). It all counts. Why? Because oxytocin, the bonding hormone, helps dial down cortisol. So being in community isn't just emotional support. It's a biological tool. We are wired to regulate together. So yes, your friend date over FaceTime or that online workout class you do with your sister is medicine. Take the dose.

Journaling isn't fluffy; it's effective.

I know, I know. Journaling sounds like something you start, forget about, and find under a pile of books three months later. Catch this: people who journal lose 50 percent more weight than those who don't. Not because writing burns calories (wouldn't that be a great workout?)—but because it interrupts autopilot.

It gives you a space to name what's hard, get all the things out of your head, own what's working, and choose what happens next. It helps you shift out of reactive mode and into conscious action.

Overthinking it? I got you. Use prompts like:

Here's what challenged me today...
Here's what I'm proud of...
Here's what I'll attempt next time...

Gratitude, reflections, frustrations—it all counts. Just make it real and actionable. And no, it doesn't have to be on paper. If typing helps you do it, go for it.

Protein + Fiber. Every. Time. You. Eat.

Stress spikes your blood sugar and creates cravings. The best counterbalance is stabilizing meals. That means quality protein and fiber every time you eat. Even your snacks. Especially your snacks.

Try:

- Carrots + hummus
- Edamame + cucumber
- Hard-boiled eggs + orange/yellow bell peppers
- Almonds + an apple
- That flourless chocolate cake from my recipe archives (yes, really)

Make it easy to do the healthful thing.

Put the nutrient-dense stuff front and center—fridge eye-level, desk-side bowls, whatever works. Put the not-so-nutritious stuff somewhere inconvenient. Like back-of-the-cabinet, behind-the-rice-cooker inconvenient. I know a woman who put all her chocolate in a mini lockbox behind all her shoes in the bottom of her closet. To which I say, whatever works. You do you.

Most importantly, this isn't about moralizing food. It's about making your defaults match your goals. The easier it is to grab the healthier option, the more likely you'll do it, especially when stress is high.

Finish the stress cycle.

When we move—walk, dance, stretch, clean the kitchen with music on—we use up the cortisol our body produced and the blood sugar coursing through our veins in case we needed to run. You don't need a gym; you just need movement. Ten minutes counts. Walking the dog counts. Dancing in your kitchen absolutely counts.

If your old routine feels impossible right now, give yourself permission to shift it. This isn't about perfection. It's about chemistry. You move your body? You help complete the stress cycle. You feel better. Period.

Permission and Practice

Look, we can't bubble-wrap ourselves from life. Work deadlines, family drama, money stuff, the news—you're never going to eliminate stress completely. That's not the goal. The goal is to stop letting it build up in your body like static electricity with nowhere to go.

You now know what stress is—a cycle your body was built to complete. You now know that cravings, fatigue, foggy thinking, and stubborn weight aren't moral failings; they're chemical responses. You now know there are real, simple ways to shift that chemistry.

Not by overhauling your life. Not by becoming some perfectly zen person who journals for two hours and does gratitude yoga under moonlight. Just by interrupting the loop. Completing the cycle. Giving your nervous system the signal that it can stand down.

So what does that look like today?

- Maybe it's breathing deep while you wait for the coffee to brew.
- Maybe it's sending your friend that meme you laughed at last night.
- Maybe it's choosing almonds instead of the leftover birthday cake.
- Maybe it's writing three lines in your notes app about what went well today.

None of these are flashy. They simply work. And when you do them consistently, they change how your body handles stress.

12

Sleep Is the Ultimate Biohack

You know that moment when you're watching someone spend $300 on a fancy supplement stack, all while living on four hours of sleep, skipping breakfast, and falling asleep with their phone on their chest? Yeah. That.

Here's the thing: A lot of us are stepping over $100 bills to pick up pennies. We're plunging ourselves into ice baths, wearing infrared masks, sipping mushroom lattes, and calling it wellness, but meanwhile, we're not sleeping. And if you're not sleeping, nothing else matters. Not really, but almost.

When I say that sleep is the ultimate biohack, I'm not being cute. I mean it in the most literal, cellular, research-backed way. Sleep is the single most powerful, most underutilized, most effective thing you can do for your health, mood, metabolism, immune system, hormones, brain function—everything you care about.

And we're ignoring it. Or worse, we're wearing sleep deprivation like a badge of honor. Bragging about how busy we are, how much we're hustling, how little we've slept. It's become the weirdest form of social currency.

Let me be blunt: No supplement can fix a lifestyle that fundamentally disrespects your body's need for rest. Sleep isn't optional. It's not a luxury. It's not weakness. It's biology.

So if you're constantly feeling like you're doing "everything right" but nothing's changing—if you're stuck in that loop of effort without results—it might be time to stop reaching for another hack and start rebuilding your base. And that starts with sleep.

Understanding Sleep

Sleep isn't a static state your body enters and exits like flipping a light switch. It's a dynamic, staged process with your brain and body cycling through multiple rounds of repair and regulation, roughly every ninety minutes.

Each cycle contains distinct phases:

- **Light sleep**, where your body begins to relax, but you can still be easily woken
- **Deep sleep**, when your physical body gets down to business repairing tissue, strengthening your immune system, and restoring cells
- **REM sleep** (Rapid Eye Movement), which is where the brain does its work: consolidating memories, regulating emotions, processing the backlog of the day

A whole night of sleep means moving through these cycles four to six times, in a relatively smooth sequence. But here's what most people don't realize: you don't spend the same amount of time in each phase throughout the night. Deep sleep tends to dominate the earlier part of the night, while REM sleep ramps up in the early morning hours. That's why disrupting sleep early versus late can have completely different effects and why consistent bedtimes matter just as much as wake times.

Also important: you want to wake up at the edge of a cycle, not in the middle of one. Ever wake up feeling foggy, heavy, and disoriented, even after a full eight hours? You may have popped awake in the middle of REM, right when your brain was still mid-download.

And yes, sleep patterns change with age. For example, people under thirty might get up to two hours of deep sleep a night; over sixty-five, that might be closer to thirty minutes. But the need for sleep, and its role in health, doesn't go away.

The idea that "more sleep = better" isn't wrong; it's just not the full picture. You need complete cycles, not just more minutes. And you need to give your body the time and consistency it needs to complete those cycles in rhythm, not fight them every night with erratic schedules and overstimulation.

The Circadian System

While your sleep cycles are driven by internal brain mechanisms (what's called homeostatic sleep pressure), they don't run on their own. They run on a schedule.

That schedule is set by your circadian system, which governs when you fall asleep, how long you stay asleep, and what kind of sleep your body prioritizes at different times of night. More deep sleep early on, more REM in the early morning—that's your rhythm.

You may have heard of circadian rhythm described as your "internal clock," which is only partially accurate because it's essentially a system of clocks. You've got a master clock in your brain, and a whole network of smaller clocks in your organs and every cell. The goal is for all of them to work in harmony, like instruments in an orchestra. Most of us? We're playing jazz at midnight with a drummer in the gut and a violinist in the pancreas, and no conductor in sight.

Your brain's master clock lives in a part of the hypothalamus called the suprachiasmatic nucleus, or SCN for short (because no one wants to say "suprachiasmatic" five times fast). This SCN is wired directly to your optic nerve, which means it gets its cue from light. Sunlight in the morning tells your body, "Hey, it's go time." Darkness at night says, "Wrap it up." That's how the rhythm starts.

But that's just the headliner. Every organ from your gut, liver, pancreas, all the way down to your fat cells, has its own local clock. These are called peripheral clocks, and they're not just waiting around for the brain's permission. They sync up based on cues like food timing, movement, and light exposure.

So when everything's working together—SCN at the top, organs playing their part—you feel energized, productive, and tired at appropriate times. You digest properly. You regulate blood sugar. You sleep deeply. You wake up with energy. When those clocks fall out of sync? It's chaos.

Imagine the mind saying, "Time for bed," while the eyes are getting daylight signals (your phone, the TV), and the pancreas is like, "Wait, we're eating now?" That mismatch between central and peripheral clocks is called circadian misalignment, and it's a recipe for metabolic dysfunction, hormone imbalances, mood swings, and more.

You don't have to be a shift worker to experience it either. One late night a week. A Netflix binge. A red-eye flight. Scrolling in bed. All of that sends mixed signals to your body's timing system. And the impact is real.

Here's a fun (and slightly gross) study: researchers looked at mice that were fed poop from other mice—don't worry, it was for science. Mice that got poop from jet-lagged mice gained more weight than those that didn't. In other words, even your microbiome knows when you've flown through time zones. Because your gut bacteria have a circadian rhythm too, and when they're off, so is everything else.

It gets wilder. The European Union defines a "shift worker" as anyone who stays awake for two to three hours between 10:00 p.m. and 5:00 a.m. at least fifty times a year. Seems like a lot until you realize that's less than once a week. (Woof!) So if you've ever said, "I'll catch up on sleep this weekend"—congratulations, you're a shift worker now.

And the fallout isn't just feeling groggy. Circadian misalignment has been linked to:

- Poor glucose tolerance
- Increased food cravings
- Mood disorders like anxiety and depression
- Hormonal disruption
- A higher risk of Type 2 diabetes and certain cancers

The body is brilliant. Yet if you constantly confuse it—feeding it late at night, skipping breakfast, blinding it with blue light at midnight—it can't do its job.

And while we all know we want to be getting a solid eight hours, it's not just about how much you sleep. It's when you sleep. Your biology is time-sensitive. Your metabolism is time-sensitive. Your hormones, your digestion, your energy—it's all running on a schedule. You don't need to control every minute. You do need to stop fighting your own clock.

Sleep Deprivation Is a Full-Body Malfunction

You might think you're just tired. But sleep deprivation doesn't show up with a name tag. It shows up as everything else. It shows up as cravings. As brain fog (ever thought: *I forgot why I walked into this room?*) It shows up as irritability, anxiety, a cold that won't go away, or gaining weight even though "nothing's changed." It shows up as that feeling of trying to function through molasses, and you can't quite name why.

Sleep loss doesn't just make you tired. It makes you less you. When you're short on sleep, your body:

- Loses sensitivity to insulin (hello, blood sugar rollercoaster)
- Increases ghrelin (your hunger hormone) and decreases leptin (your fullness hormone)
- Craves more high-glycemic, fast fuel, high-reward foods
- Struggles to process emotions and stress
- Suppresses immune function
- Messes with memory and focus

Many people don't realize their symptoms are sleep-related because the dysfunction becomes their new normal. They're not collapsing from exhaustion; they're just constantly coping. Overcaffeinating. Overeating. Overcommitting. Sound familiar?

One of the most common red flags I hear is memory issues. Clients will say things like, "I'm losing it; I can't remember anything anymore." Often, it's not a memory problem. It's an attention problem. And attention requires energy. When you're exhausted, your brain doesn't register what's happening in the first place, so there's nothing to retrieve later. No energy in, no clarity out.

Let's not forget the emotional weight of it all. When you're underslept, life feels harder. Little things become big things. You get reactive, overwhelmed, and more likely to skip workouts or grab sugar for a quick hit of energy. And the cycle repeats.

Reclaiming Your Rhythm

The good news? Sleep is fixable. Not overnight *(see what I did there?)*, but through small, intentional shifts that realign your body's internal timing system. You don't need a PhD, a $300 tracker, or a retreat in Costa Rica. You just need to get your clocks talking to each other again.

This isn't a sleep hygiene checklist. This is about understanding what your body needs to restore rhythm, starting with the basics.

1. Wake Time Is Everything

If you only do one thing after reading this chapter, let it be this: wake up at the same time every day. Yes, even on weekends. That wake time is your anchor. It trains your circadian rhythm, setting off the domino effect for the rest of your biological clocks: your appetite, your mood, your energy, and your metabolism.

Back to the symphony metaphor, if the conductor doesn't show up on time, the rest of the orchestra is just guessing. Bonus: your bedtime will fall into place when you wake at the same time each day.

2. Get Morning Light ASAP

The second-best thing you can do for sleep? Light. First thing. On your eyeballs. Don't stare at the sun. Just step outside or, at the very least, get near a window. Let that natural light hit your retinas. This simple act tells your SCN, the master clock, that it's morning. That, in turn, sets your 24-hour rhythm in motion: cortisol wakes up, melatonin goes down, metabolism kicks on, and digestion gears up. Even if it's cloudy, get outside. Natural daylight is still exponentially more effective than indoor lighting.

3. Food Tells Your Organs What Time It Is

Your first meal acts like a timestamp for your digestive system. The earlier you eat (within reason), the better your body can process that food because your insulin sensitivity is highest earlier in the day. Eating too late, on the other hand? It's like blasting a foghorn at midnight.

The sweet spot: Finish eating two to three hours before bed (three to four hours if you're in the perimenopause/menopause phase of life). Not because it's a "rule," but because your body can't multitask quality sleep and digestion. Skipping breakfast also confuses the system, especially if you're then eating most of your food at night. And, no, coffee does not count as breakfast.

4. Limit the Chaos Cues

Caffeine. Alcohol. Stress. Blue light. These are all powerful disruptors of your rhythm, and we often use them to "cope" with being tired, which only deepens the misalignment.

- **Caffeine**: Know your cutoff time. For most people, that's no later than 2:00 p.m.
- **Alcohol**: It might help you fall asleep (er, pass out), but it fragments your sleep cycles and blocks REM.
- **Blue Light**: Ditch the devices or use screen filters and night mode at a minimum. Bonus if you can switch to amber lighting and lamps in your home after sunset.

None of this has to be perfect. But if you're lying awake at 2:00 a.m. wondering why your brain is buzzing, this is likely why.

5. Build a Wind-Down Window

Your body needs a runway to land. That means you can't go from TikTok to deep sleep in three minutes. The transition matters.

Try one or two of these:

- A hot shower before bed (lowers core body temp = easier to fall asleep)
- Reading a physical book
- Journaling or mind-dumping on paper
- Guided meditation or breathing exercises
- "Sleepy girl mocktail" (a fun name for any calming beverage with magnesium or herbs—just skip the sugar bombs)

None of it has to be elaborate. The key is consistency. The body loves routine. If you wind down the same way every night, your body will start to get the message (like Pavlov's dogs).

6. Move Your Body, Time It Well

Regular movement helps regulate your rhythm, and timing matters.

- **Morning movement** boosts wakefulness, especially when paired with light.
- **Afternoon workouts** may be ideal for glucose control and injury prevention.
- **Late-night HIIT** can overstimulate some people and delay melatonin (your body's natural sleep elixir).

The best time to move is when you'll actually do it. But if you're not sleeping after your 9:00 p.m. HIIT class, now you know why.

7. Manage Stress Like It's Your Job

Because biologically, it kind of is. Chronic stress keeps cortisol elevated, which delays melatonin and scrambles your sleep cycle. It also increases nighttime waking and early morning alertness (a.k.a. "the 3:00 a.m. ping").

You don't need a monk's meditation practice. Still, daily exhale moments matter. What if you went for a walk without a podcast buzzing in your ear? Could you make mealtime a mini-digital detox? Play with breathwork, yoga, prayer, music, or petting your dog? Whatever calms your nervous system, do it.

13

Just Hug a Person

I n 2023, the U.S. Surgeon General declared that America is experiencing an epidemic of loneliness. (A fact that surprised no one who lived through the previous few years.) What *is* surprising? The health impact of that loneliness. According to the Surgeon General's report, the risks of social disconnection are equivalent to smoking fifteen cigarettes a day.

Let that land: Fifteen. A day.

That stat stopped me in my tracks. And honestly, it reframed something I'd been circling for a while. I know about the importance of community and connection. About how "we effort" trumps "me effort." But this time, it clicked in a new way. If loneliness is that dangerous, maybe connection is that powerful. Maybe hugs aren't just sweet or sentimental. They might be medicine.

So let's talk about what's happening in your body when you wrap your arms around someone (or even a teddy bear—yes, we'll get there). And why this free, touchy-feely thing you might write off as "nice" could be one of the most overlooked tools for holistic wellness.

The Side-Effects of a Hug

We tend to lump hugs into the emotional bucket, like they're a sign of affection, not a tool for health. Biologically, though, hugs flip actual switches in your body. Real ones.

Here's the short list of what gets released during a meaningful hug:

- **Oxytocin**, the "love hormone," reduces the stress response and can even lower blood pressure.
- **Dopamine**, the "pleasure hormone," gives you that "ahhh" feeling of safety or joy.
- **Serotonin**, the mood-lifting chemical that helps ease anxiety and stabilize emotions.

Together, these lower stress, reduce inflammation, and even improve cardiac function.

This isn't just feel-good fluff; this is measurable physiology. In one study of 200 adults, the group who held hands and hugged for just 20 seconds had greater drops in blood pressure and heart rate than those who simply sat together.

In another study, people with stronger support systems, measured in part by frequency of hugs, were less likely to get sick, and if they did, they had milder symptoms.

One theory? Gentle pressure on the sternum during a hug may stimulate the thymus gland, which helps regulate white blood cell production and immune response.

Another? Hugs calm the sympathetic nervous system (your fight-or-flight mode), and activate the parasympathetic nervous system (your rest, digest, recover mode) via the vagus nerve. Translation: Hugs help you stop running from lions, real or imagined, and start healing.

Hugs With Benefits

The research shows different thresholds for different benefits:

- **10-second hug:** boosts the immune system, lightens mood, eases fatigue
- **20-second hug:** reduces stress, improves heart health, calms the nervous system
- **More hugs per day = more benefit:**

  - 4 per day—survival
  - 8 per day—maintenance
  - 12 per day—growth

Don't overthink it. This isn't a checklist; it's a call to connect. And if you're not a hugger? That's okay too. Hugs with pets count. Hugging a teddy bear even showed reduced existential fear in people with low self-esteem.

You can also try a self-hug. Wrap your arms around yourself and hold for twenty seconds. Yes, really. Although, let's be clear: This isn't saying "just go hug it out" and forget about food, sleep, or movement. This isn't bypassing boundaries or ignoring discomfort around physical touch. And it's definitely not prescribing forced affection. It is saying that connection counts. And touch, when it feels safe, is a potent, often-overlooked form of nourishment.

PART III

Read the Signs

PART III

14

You Can't Supplement Your Way to Health

"*I don't believe in supplements.*"

Cool. Here's the thing: it's not a religion. Supplements exist whether you believe in them or not. This isn't about faith. It's about understanding. And most of the time, when someone says they don't believe in supplements, what they're really saying is, *I don't fully understand them, and I don't want to be sold something I don't need.*

Which, by the way, is entirely fair. The supplement world is confusing. It's crowded with flashy labels, aggressive marketing, and products that promise everything from instant energy to eternal youth. No wonder we want to shut the whole thing down.

Let's talk about the other extreme, too. The "take this and it'll fix everything" fantasy. The idea that one capsule will reset your hormones, melt your belly fat, and turn you into a glowing, zen goddess by Friday.

Have you heard someone say "there's a pill for every ill" when talking about doctors and the pharmaceutical industry? Some people take that same approach with supplements. I lovingly call them supplementarians. And also not how this works.

If you're relying on supplements to be your savior—to undo a chronically chaotic lifestyle, or to replace food, rest, and movement—you're going to be disappointed, at best. Even the most advanced formula in the world can't overrule sleep deprivation, burnout, or a vending-machine lunch.

So let's drop the belief debate altogether. Because supplements aren't miracles. They're also not scams. They're tools. And like any tool, their power depends on how, when, and why you use them.

Why Supplements Might Matter (Even If You Eat Well)

Here's a truth that wellness marketing often skips: You can't supplement your way out of poor nutrition or poor lifestyle choices. Here's another truth: You might still need to supplement with a high-quality one. Why? Because the nutritional landscape has changed, and not necessarily in our favor.

Let's start with the numbers. Around 27 percent of daily caloric intake in the US comes from calorie-rich, nutrient-poor foods. Add alcohol to that (another 4 percent), and we're looking at over 30 percent of our daily calories offering little to no nutritional value. That's one-third of your plate offering substance, but not support.

Now add in the fact that our modern produce, those fruits and vegetables we're told to load up on, often aren't as nutritious as they once were. Thanks to modern farming practices, we've got tomatoes that look perfect on the outside but are missing key minerals on the inside. Our food looks the same as what our grandparents ate, but the nutritional value has declined significantly.

Even if you're doing "everything right"—eating your plants, cutting back on processed foods, shopping the perimeter of the grocery store—you still might not be getting what your body needs to thrive. Not because you're failing, but because the system is.

And truth be told, if you eat cereal, drink milk, or have ever bought anything labeled "fortified," congratulations, you're already supplementing. If your orange juice says "with calcium," that's a supplement. If your cereal says "fortified with iron and B12," that's also a supplement. If you're drinking a protein shake or grabbing a bar that touts its vitamin content—yep, still counts.

We tend to think of supplements as little capsules in amber bottles. In reality, the idea of "supplementation" is baked into the modern food supply. It's not just something health nuts or bodybuilders do; it's something most of us are doing every day without realizing it.

Why? Because most processed foods are, well, processed. In that processing, they lose a lot of their nutritional value. So manufacturers add the nutrients back in, hence the fortification. It's a patch job on a broken system, and it's still supplementation.

That matters. Because when we say we don't *need* supplements, we're often ignoring the fact that our food already leans on them to be nutritionally adequate. And if even the food industry knows our food needs help, maybe we want to take that seriously, too.

No, this isn't a free pass to eat junk and pop a pill. It is a wake-up call. Even a decent nutrition plan might not meet all the body's needs. That's where supplementation comes in. It's in the name—supplement. To add to. To fill the gaps left by our modern food landscape and our modern lives.

Let's be clear: No pill, powder, or packet is a substitute for whole, real food.

Supplements can support you. They cannot save you from a life of drive-thru dinners, vending machine lunches, and snacks coming from bags or through windows. You cannot out-supplement a lifestyle that's missing the basics.

What People Get Wrong About Supplements

Let's bust a few myths while we're here, shall we?

Myth #1: Supplements are a replacement for healthy eating.
Nope. They're called supplements, not substitutes. They're designed to add to your nutrition, not replace it. You can't eat garbage all day and expect a capsule to fix it. That's not a wellness strategy; that's wishful thinking.

Myth #2: All supplements are the same.
Not even close. There's a massive difference between a gummy loaded with sugar and fillers and a therapeutic-grade supplement with research-backed ingredients and proper dosing. Not all formulations are created equal, and not all of them work.

Speaking of gummies—cute? Yes. Helpful? Sometimes. Many gummy vitamins are full of artificial flavors, coatings, or ingredients that interfere with absorption. Not to mention, you're often getting a fraction of the dose your body needs. (Also, trans fats in a vitamin? Come on. I've seen it! Wish it wasn't the case.)

Myth #3: Supplements aren't regulated.
This one gets thrown around a lot, usually as a reason to write off the whole category. But here's the truth: Supplements are regulated, just not in the way most people assume.

In the US, dietary supplements fall under a separate category, thanks to the Dietary Supplement Health & Education Act (DSHEA) of 1994. That law gave the FDA authority over supplement safety, manufacturing, labeling, and authorized ingredient use. The FTC also plays a role by monitoring marketing claims to protect consumers from misleading information.

So no, it's not a free-for-all out there. Companies must:

- Register their products with the FDA
- Follow Good Manufacturing Practices (GMP)
- Substantiate any health-related labeling and marketing claims
- Provide a Certificate of Analysis proving product identity, purity, potency, and limits on contaminants
- Avoid any claim that a supplement can treat, cure, or prevent disease

That last part's important: If a product claims to cure cancer or eliminate depression, it's breaking the rules. And I hope it will now set off your internal siren like it does mine.

Now, is enforcement perfect? No. Just like with food regulation, there are still bad actors, companies that cut corners or make shady claims. Regulation exists, but it's not flawless. That's why we, as consumers, still need to be discerning.

So yes, the supplement industry is regulated. And that doesn't mean you trust every bottle on a shelf. It means the smart move is working with a trusted advisor, someone who's doing the homework you don't want to do.

Myth #4: Supplements don't really work.

Well, some do and some don't. It depends on what you're taking, why you're taking it, and whether the product is actually what it claims to be.

Here's what matters:

- **Ingredient quality.** Is it the version that's been studied, or a cheap knockoff?
- **Dosage.** Are you getting enough to make a difference, or just enough to say it's in there?

- **Formulation.** Does it include the supporting nutrients needed for absorption and use? (Remember: nothing in the body works in isolation. And nothing in nature exists in isolation.)
- **Your body.** Even great supplements won't work if they're not matched to your unique needs, goals, or timing.

It's no wonder people say, "I tried supplements, and they didn't work." If you bought the wrong form, the wrong dose, or didn't give it enough time—of course it didn't work. That doesn't mean supplements are a scam. It means the execution was off.

Think of it like baking. You can have all the right ingredients, but if you use the wrong measurements, skip the baking powder, or crank the oven to 500°, you're not getting cake. You're getting regret. Yes, supplements can absolutely work. When used wisely, consistently, and with clarity.

Myth #5: Natural means safe.

Arsenic is natural. Hemlock is natural. So is mercury. Natural doesn't equal safe or effective. Read the label. Know the ingredients. And avoid anything that claims to cure something; that's a red flag (and non-DSHEA compliant).

Myth #6: I only need the one trendy ingredient I heard about on that talk show.

Ah, the Dr. Oz Effect (before Dr. Oz was in politics or worked for government agencies). Here's the problem: you remember the ingredient, but not the dose, the form, the sourcing, or the context. And the person at the store likely doesn't know either. So now you're standing in an aisle with a bottle that might be 10 percent of what you need and wondering why it's not doing anything. Because here's the thing: supplements work best when you understand what you're using and why. That's how they go from maybe helpful to truly supportive.

How to Tell If You Need Supplements

You don't need a PhD or a DNA test to start asking helpful questions. Sometimes the simplest check-in can tell you a lot. So if you're wondering, *Should I be taking supplements?*—start here:

- Do you eat processed foods?
- Do you drink alcohol?
- Do you smoke or vape?
- Are you exposed to chemicals or pollution, like city air, cleaning products, or a job that puts you in contact with toxins?
- Are you getting enough sleep?
- Do you experience stress (are you human)?
- Could you use more energy?
- Do you want to feel better than you do right now?

If you said yes to even a couple of those, supplementation might help. This doesn't mean you need to start popping pills tomorrow. It means there's reason to explore supplements, especially if you're feeling "off" and can't quite explain why.

And look, you can absolutely work with a professional (more on that in a minute), but even without testing or labs, your symptoms and lifestyle are data. If you're dragging through your day, not sleeping well, craving things constantly, or just feeling flat—that's information.

Start there. Get curious. Ask better questions. The goal isn't to diagnose yourself, it's to stop ignoring what your body is trying to tell you. Because your body is talking, and supplements might be part of how you respond.

Less is Definitely More

This is where a lot of people go sideways. You realize you might need supplements, and suddenly your bathroom looks like a mini-GNC.

Let's pause.

Supplements are powerful, but they're not Pokémon. You don't need to collect them all. Before you start buying bottles, here's the smarter move—start with your goals. What are you trying to support? Is it energy? Sleep? Hormones? Stress? Joint pain? Brain fog? Your target determines your tools. Otherwise, you're just guessing, and guessing gets expensive.

Now, can you work with your doctor? Sure. But most conventional doctors aren't trained in supplementation beyond deficiency prevention. So if you want support that goes beyond "your blood work looks fine," you'll likely want to work with someone who specializes in this space—like a Functional Diagnostic Nutrition Practitioner (FDNP), a functional medicine provider, or someone who is steeped in the industry. Every supplement is a rabbit hole, a whole world of research, dosage, quality, and bioavailability. That's why it's worth getting guidance. Not from the seventeen-year-old at the supplement store. (No shade. Just not your expert.)

And if you're not ready for testing or appointments, start smaller. Keep a simple symptom journal: How's your sleep? Your mood? Digestion? Skin? Energy? The more you notice, the more intentional you can be. Awareness is step one. Strategy is step two.

You Can't Trust the Price Tag

Here's a hard truth in the supplement world: You can't trust the price tag to tell you what's quality support. Cheaper doesn't always mean worse. Expensive doesn't always mean better. And sometimes the $9.99 multivitamin on sale is just expensive pee.

So how do you know what you're getting? Let's break it down.

A high-quality supplement checks these boxes:

- **Clinically evidenced ingredients.** Are they the forms of nutrients that your body can use? (Not all magnesium or B12 is created equal.)

- **Effective dose.** Are you getting enough of the ingredient to do something? Many brands sprinkle a trendy nutrient in there just so they can list it on the label, but not at a clinically effective dose.
- **Supporting cast.** Is that key ingredient paired with the nutrients it needs to work? (Remember: nutrients don't operate solo; they need other nutrients to unlock their superpowers.)
- **Clean formulation.** Look for minimal fillers, artificial colors, flavors, or coatings. You don't need carcinogens or trans fats in your multivitamin.

And this is where working with someone who knows their stuff helps. Because let's be honest: you don't have time to become a supplement sourcing expert. That's not your job. But it is your right to know that what you're taking is actually helping, not just sitting in your cabinet collecting dust (or worse, causing harm).

Omega-3s are a perfect example. The quality ones? Game-changing. The other ones? Rancid, contaminated, and often dosed so low you'd need to take fifteen doses a day just to see results.

Yes, ask questions. Do your research. And if all else fails, find someone who can help you filter the noise. Because in supplements, as in life, quality matters more than quantity.

Women's Health Is a Moving Target

If you're looking for a one-size-fits-all supplement for women, stop. It doesn't exist. Why? Because women's bodies are dynamic. Like, really dynamic. Your hormones, energy, and nutrient needs shift, not just over the decades, but literally every single day.

You're not just dealing with "female hormones." You're dealing with thirty-day biochemical choreography that affects everything from your mood to your metabolism. Add stress, sleep, toxins, body composition, and aging into the mix, and you start to see why no bottle labeled "Women's Health" can possibly cover it all.

What works during PMS won't necessarily work during menopause. What supports fertility might not be what your body needs during perimenopause. It's not random; it's rhythmic. And it requires attention. What does that mean for supplements?

It means:

- Focus on balance over silver bullets
- Support your system as a whole—energy, sleep, stress, detox—not just estrogen or progesterone
- Your phase of life matters (are you menstruating, postpartum, perimenopausal, postmenopausal?)
- Your lifestyle matters (are you sleeping? Managing stress? Moving your body?)

If you're looking for a place to start, focus on foundational support: nutrients that impact energy, brain health, detoxification, and resilience. And yes, that might include herbs or hormone-adjacent support, but always in context, and ideally, with expert guidance.

Bottom line? Your needs as a woman are specific, real, and continually evolving. So skip the random recommendations and start with where you are.

The Starting Lineup

Let's say you're cautiously willing to dip a toe in the supplement world, and you're asking, *Where do I start?*

If I had to choose just three supplements to recommend to most people (and yes, I hesitate to be prescriptive with this because this stuff is personal), here's my foundational lineup:

1. **A High-Quality Multivitamin.** Look for one that includes a B-complex, vitamin D3, and chromium. Think of this as your daily insurance policy, covering a broad base of

nutritional needs, especially for energy, metabolism, and immunity.

2. **Magnesium.** Most people are deficient, especially women. Magnesium supports muscle relaxation, sleep, blood pressure, mood, and over 300 bodily functions (possibly more). Look for forms like magnesium citrate or glycinate; they're easier for your body to absorb. Bonus if it includes potassium, too.

3. **Omega-3 Fatty Acids.** Specifically, DHA and EPA from deep-sea fish like sardines or anchovies (not salmon or tuna, which can be high in mercury). These support heart health, brain function, inflammation, skin, and more. Check the dose; you want 3,000 mg for general support. And make sure it's cold-pressed, sourced in the US, and doesn't repeat on you. (Pro tip: Freeze it. If it doesn't freeze solid, that's a good sign.)

Are these the only quality, supportive options? No. Are they a smart, evidence-based place to start for most people? Yes. But again, start with what you notice in your body. Then layer in support one smart step at a time.

How to Track What's Working (Without Losing Your Mind)

So you've started a supplement. Now what? How do you know if it's working? How long do you wait? Should you keep a journal? Use an app? Create a color-coded Excel sheet with bar graphs? Here's my take: Keep it simple, or you won't do it. You don't need a fancy system.

This could be:

- A quick note in your phone
- A sentence in your planner
- A sticky note on the bathroom mirror

Write down what you're taking and what you notice. Are you sleeping better? Less bloated? Less cranky? More clear-headed? Are your workouts easier? Is your energy more stable? If you're working with a practitioner, they might give you a whole spreadsheet to track symptoms and timing. And if that works for you? Great. But if you're like a lot of us, that spreadsheet lasts maybe a day. You need something that fits into real life.

And when it comes to timing, here's a good rule of thumb:

- Start one supplement at a time
- Wait at least three days, ideally a week or two, before adding another
- If you feel something shift—positive or negative—note it

This isn't about turning into a supplement scientist. It's about building self-awareness. Noticing patterns. Giving your body the space and time to respond. You deserve better than throwing capsules at the wall to see what sticks. And your body deserves the kind of attention that helps you figure out what's truly helping.

The Bottom Line on Supplements

Let's land the plane. You cannot supplement your way out of poor nutrition. You also can't ignore how modern life creates real gaps, even with quality nutrition. Supplements aren't the enemy. They're not a miracle. They're a tool.

Used intentionally, they can support your energy, sleep, stress, hormones, digestion, cognition, and overall vitality. Used reactively, randomly, or recklessly, they can waste your money, give you false hope, create even more confusion, or potentially cause health challenges.

So what's the path?

1. **Start with your goals.**
   What are you looking to support—mood, metabolism, joint health, hormonal balance?

2. **Get your foundation in place.**
   That means food, sleep, movement, and stress. Supplements can't fix what your lifestyle is constantly breaking.

3. **Layer in support slowly.**
   One thing at a time. Pay attention. Adjust as you go.

4. **Work with an expert if you can.**
   Someone who knows what questions to ask and what signs to watch for.

5. **Trust your body.**
   It's not broken. It just might need backup.

In the end, this isn't about doing everything "right." It's about figuring out what works—for you, in your life—with a little science, a little curiosity, and a whole lot of self-compassion.

15

Let's Talk About Sex, Baby

I f Salt-N-Pepa taught us anything, it's that talking about sex is never just about sex.

It's about what's working. What's not. And all the good things and the bad things that may be. So, let's talk about sex. (Go ahead, try not to sing it—I'll wait.)

But seriously, we don't talk about sex, so it's no surprise that we don't talk about, well—*not* having it. You used to want it. Now, not so much. Or not at all. Maybe it takes forever to get in the mood. Maybe the mood never even shows up. And part of you wonders: *Is this just what getting older feels like? Is it hormones? Stress? My relationship? Am I just—broken?*

Let me assure you, you're not broken. You are missing real information. The truth is that your sex drive doesn't just vanish out of nowhere. It drops for a reason (or ten). And most of them are things no one's ever connected for you. Things like poor sleep. Chronic stress. Cardiovascular health. Blood sugar rollercoasters. Meds. Mood.

We're told to treat libido like a mood ring. But it's more like a dashboard light. When your sex drive tanks, it's often not just about sex. It's your body flagging that something's off under the hood. This chapter is here to connect the dots no one else is talking about. Not to make your sex life a project (we all know you don't need more of those), but to make it make sense.

So yeah, we're going there.

Libido is a System

Here's what most people don't realize: Your libido is a system, not a setting. It's not just hormones. It's not just how attracted you are. It's not just an age thing. It's an equation made up of blood flow, stress load, sleep quality, metabolic function, nervous system tone, nutrient status, relationship dynamics, and, yep, hormones. Which means: if any one of those pieces is struggling, sex is going to slide down the priority list. Not because you're not into it. But because your body is busy surviving, not thriving.

Let's break down the big players:

Stress

Stress is a libido killer. And no, not just the bad kind. Any constant mental load keeps your nervous system in a state that says, *Now is not the time to get naked.* Why? Because stress raises cortisol. And chronically high cortisol suppresses sex hormones. It also tanks your energy, kills your sleep, and tells your brain that pleasure is non-essential. Remember, the body's stress response is designed to keep us alive. Procreating doesn't matter if we aren't alive in the twenty minutes to do it. (Yes, do it.)

Sleep

Sleep is your body's nightly hormone reset. Without enough of it, testosterone, estrogen, and progesterone get scrambled.

Libido drops. Energy tanks. Mood follows. That glass of wine you think is helping you unwind? It's sedating you, not giving you quality, restorative sleep. You don't wake up refreshed. You wake up depleted and disinterested.

Blood Flow

For arousal to happen, you need adequate blood flow to your sex organs. If you've got high blood pressure, poor circulation, or elevated blood sugar, that's not happening. And no, it's not just a "guy thing." Women need blood flow, too—for lubrication, for sensitivity, for literally feeling something. Medications for blood pressure, cholesterol, and depression can also tank libido and interfere with orgasm. You're not imagining it.

Hormones

For women, shifts in estrogen, progesterone, and testosterone (especially during perimenopause) influence desire. The bigger story is how those hormones are being impacted by everything else: stress, nutrition, movement, and sleep. For men, everyone loves to blame testosterone. But less than 10 percent of male sexual dysfunction is caused by low testosterone. Over 70 percent is linked to blood sugar dysfunction and cardiovascular issues (blood flow).

What Your Sexual Health Is Telling You

Let's simplify what your libido is telling you: Low desire is often just low bandwidth. When you're underslept, overstressed, nutrient-depleted, and running on caffeine and cortisol, sex becomes one more thing on a list you're already drowning under. Of course, it drops off.

This isn't about "getting your mojo back" with a smoothie or some sexy lingerie. This is about giving your body what it needs to feel safe, energized, and responsive. Here's the mental filter: Sexual health is a downstream indicator.

It reflects how your upstream systems are functioning:

- Are you sleeping?
- Are you moving?
- Are you eating for blood sugar balance?
- Are you recovering from stress, or always layering more on?

When those systems improve, libido tends to follow. Get curious. Play with some of these and notice how you feel.

Replace the wine wind-down with magnesium (glycinate and citrate) or a warm bath a few nights a week. Notice if your sleep deepens, and if your mood (or interest) shifts the next day or over time.

Eat for blood flow. Add dark leafy greens, beets, berries, and healthful fats like salmon. These support nitric oxide, which supports circulation, which supports arousal. Yes, food foreplay is a thing.

Build muscle. Just a couple of strength training sessions a week can shift hormone production, improve insulin sensitivity, and boost confidence—all of which show up in the bedroom.

Guard your sleep like it matters. Because it does. No screen-scrolling in bed. No over-caffeinating to push through. Give yourself seven to nine hours of what your hormones are begging for.

You don't need to do everything. Noticing which inputs are helping, and which ones are quietly stealing your spark, is powerful. And remember, when you manage the stress, you make space for the sex.

16

Poop Is a Vital Sign

Let's just say it—poop. There. We survived.

If you're already squirming, that's kind of the point. We've been trained to treat this part of life like it's shameful, embarrassing, or somehow beneath the conversation. The truth is that poop is one of the most honest indicators of your health. It's daily feedback from your body, and most of us are too busy holding it in—literally and figuratively—to listen.

This chapter isn't about making you obsessed with every trip to the bathroom. It's about helping you understand why poop is worth noticing, what it can tell you, and how to use that information without spiraling into panic or perfectionism.

Paying attention is not the same thing as pathologizing. You don't need to diagnose yourself every time you flush. But you do need to know what's normal for you and what's not.

What Poop Is Made Of

Let's zoom out for a second and start with a simple question: what is poop? Sure, we know it as "waste," but that word doesn't do it justice. Your poop is a fascinating, complex mix of biological material—less garbage chute, more status report. It's your body's way of saying, *Here's everything I don't need. Here's how I'm functioning. Here's what I'm clearing out so I can keep running efficiently.*

In a healthy bowel movement, about 75 percent is water. Yep, mainly water. The remaining 25 percent is a blend of:

- Bacterial biomass (both dead and alive)
- Undigested food particles—often fiber that your body can't absorb
- Fat and protein residues
- Bile
- Sloughed-off intestinal cells
- Metabolic waste
- Trace toxins, microplastics, and environmental debris your body didn't absorb (yes, sadly, that includes bits from packaging, air pollution, and cosmetics)

Let that sink in. That daily visit to the toilet? It's not just the end of digestion. It's part of your body's detox system. Forget the Instagram cleanses. This is the real one. And here's where it gets more interesting. Poop is not just a report card for what you ate last night. It reflects your gut microbiome, those trillions of bacteria that live in your digestive tract and help manage everything from immunity to mood to inflammation. Scientists can analyze stool samples and detect markers for conditions like Parkinson's, autism, Crohn's, IBS, obesity, and even mental health issues. Your gut is that central. Your poop is that revealing.

Archaeologists in Denmark once uncovered an ancient latrine and studied the microbiomes of people who lived centuries ago. What did they find? Those ancient guts were more diverse than ours—more types of bacteria, better resilience. Today, our micro-biomes are less diverse and more fragile, thanks to antibiotics, processed food, and environmental toxins. And you can see that shift right in the toilet bowl.

The next time you're tempted to dismiss your poop as "gross waste," remember, it's telling a bigger story. One about how your body is processing the world, what it's managing to let go of, and where it might be holding on. You don't need to analyze every trip to the bathroom like a lab tech. But understanding what's in there helps you know what your body is doing and what it might need help with.

Read the Signs

Now that we know what poop is made of and why it matters, let's talk about what it's saying. Because once you stop looking at elimination as something gross or embarrassing, you realize that this isn't just a bodily function. It's a feedback loop. And just like any constructive feedback, it comes in a few different forms. Let's break them down.

A quick aside before we get into all that: remember, every elimination is a new elimination. Let's not judge your entire gut health based on one trip to the toilet.

Frequency: How Often Should You Go?

Let's start with the big question everyone asks: *How often should I be pooping?* The unsatisfying-but-true answer is—it depends.

There's a broad standard range, anything from three times a day to three times a week. But let's be honest, if you're only going a couple times a week, you probably don't feel great. You're likely bloated, sluggish, maybe even a little foggy. That's your body's way of telling you it wants more movement.

Ideally, your body would eliminate once per meal. Think about a baby. They eat; they poop. That's a sign of a well-functioning digestive tract. As adults, we lose that pattern for a bunch of reasons—nutrition, stress, dehydration, lack of fat or fiber, hormones, and even holding it because we're not comfortable going in public.

(Yes, we're going there. If you've ever pretended you just went in to fix your hair so you could wait until your coworker left the bathroom, I see you.)

But here's the thing: Holding it not only feels terrible, it also trains your body to stop responding to its signals. Your colon starts to stretch, weakening the muscle tone and making elimination more difficult in the future. It's a vicious cycle, and it's way more common among women. We've been taught to be polite instead of responsive.

And when you don't go, the consequences are real. Your body starts reabsorbing the waste it was intending to eliminate. That's not just uncomfortable, it's inflammatory. It affects your skin, your energy, and your immune function. And over time, it can contribute to chronic conditions.

Want to test your own transit time? Try the corn or beet test (yes, really). Eat a noticeable amount of corn or beets, then watch for when it shows up in your stool. It's your body's version of a timestamp.

Consistency: The Texture Tells a Story

If frequency is the "how often," consistency is the "how it feels." Here's your rule of thumb: We want your poop to be formed, soft, and easy to pass. No straining, no discomfort, no suspense.

Too hard? You're likely not getting enough water, fiber, or fat. Your stool sits in your colon too long, water gets reabsorbed, and suddenly you're dealing with dry, difficult, pellet-like stool. Not fun.

Too soft or watery? That could mean food sensitivities, infections, medications, or not enough fiber to bulk things up. And if it's happening frequently, your body may not be absorbing nutrients well, leading to fatigue, brain fog, or even malnutrition.

What you're aiming for is something that holds together but isn't rigid. A little like a ripe banana, not too green, not too mushy. (Yes, I know. Sorry, not sorry for that visual.)

And if you're wondering how to gauge it? Listen for the splash. The Olympic diver metaphor applies—clean entry, minimal drama.

Size and Shape: Enter the Bristol Stool Scale

I once heard the phrase "fluffy floaters, not stinker sinkers," and while that's not exactly scientific, it's not far off. Light, well-formed stools are a sign your gut is working efficiently. And yes, there's an actual scale for this. It's called the Bristol Stool Scale, and it's the bathroom equivalent of a mood ring.

It categorizes poop into seven types:

- **Type 1:** Tiny, hard pellets—definitely constipated
- **Type 2:** Lumpy and sausage-like—also constipated
- **Type 3:** Like a sausage with cracks—getting better
- **Type 4:** Smooth and snake-like—chef's kiss, this is your colon in 3D
- **Type 5:** Soft blobs with distinct edges—still solid, often from high-fiber intake
- **Type 6:** Mushy with ragged edges—bordering on diarrhea
- **Type 7:** Watery, no solid pieces—classic diarrhea

Your sweet spot is between Type 3 and Type 5. If you're consistently Type 1 or 2, add water, fat, and fiber. If you're hovering around Type 6 or 7, consider food sensitivities, hydration, and stress, and talk to your doctor if it doesn't resolve. And yes, it can vary day to day. You might have a solid morning and a softer afternoon. That's natural, and your job is to figure out if it's normal for you.

Also worth noting: size matters. Bigger movements typically mean more fiber and better gut motility. Smaller ones, or ones that come with urgency but little output, may indicate inflammation or poor transit.

There's even research that ties stool weight to disease risk. In one study, populations with low daily poop weight (around four ounces) had significantly higher rates of colon cancer. The takeaway? When you go more and go well, you're protecting your long-term health, not just enjoying momentary relief.

Color: The Crayola Box of Gut Health

Brown is the classic. That's thanks to bile, bacteria, and the breakdown of red blood cells.

Here's what other colors might mean:

- **Green:** Probably something you ate—spinach, matcha, or chlorophyll supplements. No panic.
- **Red/Maroon:** Often beets, cranberries, or red dye. But if it's actual blood in the stool, call your doc.
- **Black:** Could be iron supplements or upper GI bleeding. Pay attention, especially if paired with dizziness or fatigue.
- **Yellow:** Undigested fat, could be a gallbladder or pancreatic issue or just a super fatty meal.
- **Gray or white:** Usually a result of medical testing (like barium). Not typical otherwise.
- **Multi-colored confetti:** Maybe ease up on the artificial food dyes.

One weird color after a new recipe isn't a crisis. But if something stays off, and especially if it's paired with other symptoms, it's worth checking in.

Smell: Know Your Brand

Let's get real—poop smells. It's supposed to. But if the smell becomes especially foul, metallic, or just different than your usual, it could be telling you something. Malabsorption issues, infections, or imbalances in your gut flora can all change the scent. The goal isn't odorlessness, it's consistency. You know your baseline. If that changes and stays changed, take note.

What Impacts How You Go

If you've ever traveled, gotten sick, changed your food choices, had your period, taken antibiotics, or just had a stressful week, you've probably noticed your poop shift in response. Maybe you got constipated after a long flight. Maybe you had urgent diarrhea the day of a big presentation. Maybe your cycle hit, and suddenly things moved fast (or not at all).

None of that is random. Poop changes because your body is responsive. Let's unpack some of the most common factors that can mess with your elimination, and more importantly, what you can do about them.

1. **Fiber (And Yes, Type and Amount Matter)**
Fiber is your digestive system's MVP. But not all fiber is created equal.

Insoluble fiber adds bulk and helps move things through. Think carrots, cauliflower, dark leafy greens, green beans, nuts, and seeds.

Soluble fiber helps absorb water and slows things down. Think oats, beans, apples, barley, and Brussels sprouts.

Too little fiber = constipation. Too much, too fast = gas, bloating, or diarrhea.

Aim for 25 to 35 grams a day, mostly from fruits and vegetables. And work up to it because your gut needs time to adjust.

Bonus: Fiber also feeds your healthy gut bacteria, which helps balance your entire microbiome and nourishes the ecosystem that makes going possible.

2. **Water: Fiber's BFF**
Fiber without water is like a car without gas. It just sits there. Your stool is supposed to be 75 percent water. If you're

not drinking enough, especially when increasing fiber, things dry out, harden, and stall. Start with the classic guideline: 8 cups (64 oz) of water a day. Adjust upward if you're active, sweating, flying, or just need a little extra help getting things moving.

And no, coffee doesn't count. Yes, it might help you go (thank you, caffeine), but it's also a diuretic. So if you're relying on your morning latte to kickstart your bowels, make sure you're also chasing it with water. Or better yet, water first and then coffee.

3. Fat: The Underrated Lubricant

Let's give fat some love. For those of us raised during the low-fat diet craze, this can feel counterintuitive. But fat is essential for digestion and elimination. It lubricates the digestive tract and helps soften stool. Without enough fat, your poop might feel like it's hitting speed bumps on the way out.

One of my clients, Yana, had struggled with bowel movements for as long as she could remember, and she'd come to rely on a specific tea to help things along. Then she went to visit her sister in Florida and left the tea at home. The weather was gorgeous. Her digestion? Completely stalled.

So we checked in. Was she hydrating? Eating vegetables? Getting in enough fat? That last one caught her off guard. "What do you mean, more fat?"

We talked about what quality fat looks like—like avocado, olive oil, nuts—and how much matters. A proper serving of avocado isn't a polite slice; it's half the avocado. We also talked about spreading fat throughout the day, not just tacking it on at dinner.

A few days later, she sent me her food tracking sheet. Next to one day's lunch, she'd written: "Half an avocado with lunch and MAGIC (in all caps) happened." That afternoon, she went again. Twice in one day, without the tea. For the first time in years, her body worked without struggle.

We could all use a little of that magic in our lives, am I right? What counts? Avocados, olive oil, nuts, seeds, and full-fat yogurt if dairy works for you.

4. Movement: The Physical Kind

Your digestive system relies on peristalsis, a wave-like muscle movement, to move food through your gut. And one of the best ways to support that process? Moving your body. Walking, twisting yoga poses, dancing in your kitchen—anything that gets your blood flowing and your body moving helps stimulate digestion. Even a quick set of squats or stretching before bed can make a difference. Stillness breeds stagnation. Movement breeds movement.

5. Stress: The Silent Constipator (or Accelerator)

Stress affects everything, including your gut.

The connection between your brain and digestive tract (via the vagus nerve) means that what you feel emotionally, you also feel physically. That's why stress can either shut down digestion (leading to constipation) or accelerate it (leading to diarrhea). And it works both ways: if your gut is off, your mood often follows.

What helps? Breathwork. Sleep. Gentle movement. Saying no to the thing you don't want to do. (This one hits hard.) Reducing your stress doesn't have to mean a weeklong spa retreat. Sometimes it's just making a tiny choice that tells your nervous system, *We're safe.*

6. Medications and Supplements

Many common medications can disrupt digestion:

- Antibiotics wipe out gut bacteria (good and bad), leading to an imbalance
- Painkillers and antacids often cause constipation
- Antidepressants, antihistamines, and iron supplements can slow motility

That doesn't mean you must stop taking them, but it does mean you want to pay attention and support your gut accordingly. If you're on antibiotics, consider taking probiotics (preferably ones that survive to the correct part of the gut) and adding fermented foods and fiber to help rebuild balance. And read your labels because some "wellness" products (including protein shakes and fiber powders) can cause more harm than help if you're not careful with quality, quantity, or timing.

7. Food Sensitivities and Digestive Conditions

Sometimes poop changes aren't about a missing nutrient; they're a reaction.

Common culprits:

- Dairy (especially in those with lactose intolerance)
- Gluten
- Artificial sweeteners (sorbitol and others can cause bloating or loose stool)
- FODMAPs (a category of fermentable carbs for those with IBS)

You don't need to run out and do an elimination diet after one weird poop. But if you notice consistent patterns—like every time you eat ice cream, things go south (pun intended)—that's worth noting.

8. Travel, Sleep, Hormones, and Aging

Your bowel is a creature of habit. Disrupt its routine, and it gets cranky.

- Travel changes time zones, movement, meals, and hydration—all key for regularity.
- Sleep impacts your circadian rhythm, which helps regulate digestion.
- Menstrual cycles shift hormones like progesterone, which can slow down or speed up transit.
- Aging can lead to slower digestion, reduced physical activity, and decreased fluid intake.

None of this is cause for alarm; it is cause for awareness. If you're backed up on vacation or things shift during your period, that's biological data to pay attention to, not a sign that your body is broken. You can support your system by packing fiber-rich snacks, drinking extra water on planes, stretching after long travel days, or simply being kind to yourself when your cycle hits.

Your New Bathroom Intelligence

Poop isn't just something that happens to you. It's something your body does, and it's worth learning how to read the signals it sends. But let's be clear: you don't need to turn into a bathroom biochemist. This isn't about analyzing your stool like you're reading tea leaves or logging every detail in an app (unless you want to, in which case, no judgment).

There's a middle ground between ignoring your body entirely and obsessing over every blip. That middle ground is called awareness. Awareness is what helps you notice changes before they become problems. It's what connects the dots between what you eat, how you live, and how you feel. And it's the key to building body literacy, the kind of grounded knowing that lets you trust yourself again.

Here's how to start:

Know Your Normal

We've said it before, and we'll say it again—normal is a spectrum. Your job isn't to hit someone else's target; it's to understand your own pattern. Are you usually a once-a-day person? Do you lean toward Type 4 on the Bristol Stool Scale? Does your stool change the week before your period, or after you travel, or when you're stressed? That's your baseline. Knowing it is powerful. Because when something shifts, you'll have context. A random bout of diarrhea isn't the same as a month of inconsistency. A single green stool after a smoothie isn't the same as persistent pale poop. When you know your baseline, you're better able to spot changes that matter and ignore the ones that don't.

Look for Patterns, Not Perfection

One "off" poop is not a crisis. Even a few off days might just be your body adjusting to something new. What you want to watch for is persistence.

- Has something changed for more than a week?
- Is this happening every time you eat a particular food?
- Are you starting to feel symptoms beyond digestion—fatigue, skin issues, headaches, mood dips?

If yes, then it's worth a deeper look. But please don't spiral into overcorrection. You don't need to cut ten foods or overhaul your life after one bad bathroom trip. Your gut isn't a saboteur. It's a communicator. And often, small shifts (like more fiber, more water, or simply going when you need to go) are enough to get things back on track.

Track (If You Need To)

If something feels off and you can't figure out why, tracking can help. But keep it simple. You don't need a full diagnostic spreadsheet. Just jot a few notes in your phone or planner:

- What you ate
- How you felt
- What your poop was like (you can even code it—nobody needs to see "diarrhea" on your calendar)

This is especially helpful for symptoms that show up with a delay. Some food sensitivities (like gluten or dairy) can take days to cause issues. Same with hormonal shifts. Without a record, your brain will default to recency bias: "It must have been the eggs I ate an hour ago." Probably not. Tracking helps you see patterns over time, which is where the truth lives.

Talk to Your Doctor (Even If They Don't Ask)

If your symptoms persist or you just have questions, say something. Don't wait for your provider to bring it up. Yes, it might feel awkward. But you're not being dramatic. You're being proactive. And if your provider brushes it off? That's not a reflection on your body, but it might be a sign to find a better partner in your care.

Train Your Gut Like a Pro

Consistency isn't just for gym schedules. Your digestive system thrives on rhythm and routine. Here's how to support it:

- **Go when you need to.** Don't hold it in. Delaying trains your body to ignore its signals, and makes it harder to go when you do want to.
- **Build a ritual.** Try sitting on the toilet at the same time each day, especially in the morning or after meals, when your body is naturally more primed to eliminate.
- **Use gravity.** Squatting straightens your rectum and makes elimination easier. A squatty potty works wonders, but so will a stack of books or a flipped-over trash can.
- **Let coffee help, but hydrate.** Caffeine stimulates the bowels, but it's also dehydrating. Pair it with water to avoid setting yourself up for constipation.
- **Be patient. Be kind. Be consistent.** You're not forcing your body into compliance. You're inviting it into rhythm. With time, your gut will start responding more predictably.

Body literacy doesn't mean you track every toilet visit. It means you learn to listen. To trust your own data. To respond instead of react. Think collaboration instead of micromanagement. And like any supportive relationship, your body's asking, *Are you paying attention?*

What's Wrong with Poop Talk

At this point, you might be thinking, *Okay, I get it. Poop matters. But why are we all so weird about it?* Excellent question. Let's talk about that. The real problem with poop isn't physiological. It's cultural.

We've built a world where people will spend $60 on gut health supplements but feel embarrassed to say the word "constipated." We'll track our macros, close our rings, and DM our trainer every time we hit a new PR, but when our poop is off, we don't say a word. Not to our friends, not to our doctors, and sometimes not even to ourselves.

If you've ever held in a bowel movement because you didn't want to go in a public restroom, or delayed going until the house was empty, or flushed twice to muffle the sound, you're not alone. You're human. You've been trained and trained well. You've been taught that elimination is gross. That it's something to be ashamed of. That it's inappropriate to talk about or even acknowledge.

But guess what? Every single person you know—every coworker, every best friend, every parent at school pickup—poops. Not one of us is exempt. Your boss? Poops. Your favorite Instagram wellness coach? Poops. The person you're dating? Definitely poops.

And when we treat that basic fact of biology like it's taboo, we create distance from ourselves and each other. We cut off an important line of communication from our body. We delay getting help. We miss the signals until it's too late.

Colorectal cancer is now one of the most common cancers in the US, and rates are rising in people under fifty. Many of these cases are caught late, not because people weren't having symptoms, but because they didn't talk about them. Or their doctors didn't ask. Or they were told it was "just IBS" or "probably something you ate." We can't change what we don't talk about.

And talking about poop doesn't mean we make it the center of every conversation (in fact, please don't). It just means we normalize it. We treat it like the vital sign it is. We remove the shame so that people can ask questions, get support, and trust their bodies again.

You don't have to start giving TED Talks about your bowel movements. But here are a few ways to normalize poop in your world:

- Notice what your body is doing; don't ignore the signs
- Mention digestive shifts to your doctor, even if they don't ask
- Talk to your kids about what's normal and what's not
- Make it okay for your partner, your friend, or yourself to say, "I feel off"
- Laugh about it when it's funny; take it seriously when it's not

You don't have to be a poop evangelist. But know that every time we talk about this stuff without flinching, we chip away at the shame and permit someone else to listen to their body, too.

PART IV

But What About...

By now, you've got the big picture. You know the principles that matter most, and hopefully you feel a little less pressure to "do everything right." And sometimes the questions keeping us up at night are the nitty-gritty ones; the ones that feel urgent when you're scrolling at 11:00 p.m. or staring into the fridge.

This book is about *uncomplicating* wellness, so I don't want to overwhelm you with facts and data. I also don't want to leave you hanging. Think of this like a lightning round: What's true, what's hype, and what matters without the fluff or fear tactics.

These are the questions I get in my DMs, in line at Trader Joe's, and on coaching calls every single week. The ones people whisper like they're confessing to a crime: *Do I have to give up coffee to be healthy? Can I justify a cheat day? Are GLP-1 meds my best option?* Don't think of this as gospel, just a dose of clarity to help tame the chaos.

...fiber powders and fiber supplements?

Fiber supplements can help if you're falling short, but they're not a free pass to skip real food. Whole fruits, vegetables, legumes, and grains bring fiber plus vitamins, minerals, and phytonutrients you won't get from a scoop of powder. If you choose to use one, opt for a high-quality option with multiple sources of fiber, free from unnecessary fillers or sweeteners, and drink plenty of water to prevent digestive issues. They are not all created equal. Think of fiber powders/supplements as a backup plan, not the foundation of your fiber intake.

...coffee and caffeine?

Coffee isn't evil, or a cure-all. It can boost focus and metabolism, and too much or too late in the day can disrupt sleep, stress your adrenals, and interfere with vitamin and mineral absorption. Stick to one to two cups earlier in the day and not before food, pair each cup with water, and skip the sugar-loaded versions. If you take vitamins, have them before coffee, and consider a short caffeine break a couple of times a year to reset your system.

...cold plunges?

Cold plunges can be great for recovery and resilience. Timing is everything. Doing them first thing in the morning spikes cortisol (already naturally high) and can throw off your body's clock, leaving you wired at night and fatigued during the day. Instead, aim for post-workout or late afternoon when cortisol is lower, to boost recovery and improve sleep.

...laughter?

Turns out the cliché is true: laughter really is powerful medicine. Laughing boosts oxygen intake, stimulates your heart and lungs, and triggers endorphins that relieve stress. It can also improve circulation, lower blood pressure, and even support your immune system. Kids laugh up to 400 times a day, while adults average just 15, so we could all use more. Watch a comedy, play a silly game with friends, or even fake a laugh. (It works!) The more you laugh, the better you feel.

...eggs?

Eggs are a complete protein and rich in nutrients like choline. The cholesterol in eggs has minimal impact on blood cholesterol for most people; how the egg is cooked matters more (runny yolk or soft-cooked beats overcooked hard yolks). Unless your doctor advises otherwise, eggs can be a healthful staple.

...breakfast?

Skipping breakfast or having just coffee sends stress signals to your body and can tank energy, hormones, and thyroid function. A protein-rich breakfast (four to six ounces) within an hour of waking sets your blood sugar and cortisol on track (of course, with fiber too). If you can't eat much, try at least two to three ounces of protein, a snack size, about two eggs with maybe some carrot sticks, and then plan a mid-morning snack or proper meal, to keep blood sugar stable, prevent the afternoon crash, and late-night cravings.

...alcohol?

We get healthier each day we keep alcohol away. Alcohol is a toxin your liver prioritizes above everything else, meaning fat and sugar metabolism pause until the alcohol is processed out. That's why drinking can stall progress toward other health goals and leave you feeling sluggish. If you're going to drink (I do), keep it moderate, pair it with lighter whole foods (not sugar bombs), and hydrate well—your liver will thank you.

...non-alcoholic beer and wine?

Non-alcoholic options usually still contain up to 0.5 percent alcohol (unless labeled alcohol-free at 0 percent), which is minimal but worth noting if you're avoiding alcohol. Many beer alternatives have relatively clean ingredients. Wines can come with added sugar or sulfites to replace what's lost in processing. If you enjoy them, read the labels, compare sugar content, and choose the brands with the simplest ingredient lists.

...GMOs, bioengineered labels, and going organic or local?

GMO (genetically modified organism) foods are now often labeled as "BE" (bioengineered), and the rules have loopholes, which means heavily processed ingredients and certain gene-editing techniques don't have to be disclosed. Choosing organic or Non-GMO Project verified products is the simplest way to avoid them, and local foods often skip heavy processing altogether. If these foods are out of your budget or not available at the moment, no problem! Let's not make perfection the enemy of progress. Don't stress over every label, simply know that fresh, whole foods with minimal packaging are your safest bet.

...SIBO?

If you feel fine in the morning but look six months pregnant by evening, SIBO might be the culprit. It happens when bacteria overgrow in the small intestine, feeding on fermentable foods (high-FODMAP foods) and producing gas. Other symptoms include bloating, constipation or diarrhea, reflux, or unexplained fatigue. If this is you, don't just self-eliminate foods forever—see a gastroenterologist or functional practitioner and ask for a SIBO breath test (hydrogen, methane, or hydrogen sulfide). Treating SIBO can include targeted antibiotics (like rifaximin) or herbal antimicrobials. The goal is to reset your gut so you can return to a full, balanced nutrition plan rather than avoiding whole food groups long-term.

Also, SIBO isn't the only reason one might experience these symptoms, despite what social media and headlines will have you believe. That's why testing before eliminating foods is helpful.

...plant-based meat alternatives?

Products like Impossible and Beyond Burgers are highly processed foods designed to taste like meat. They're made with genetically modified ingredients, refined oils, and additives—not exactly the whole-food upgrade they're marketed as. If you eat meat, a grass-fed organic burger is likely a better choice; if you're vegetarian, focus on true whole-food proteins like beans, lentils, tofu, or tempeh.

...sitting, is it the new smoking?

Sitting all day is as damaging to your health as it sounds. Long stretches of inactivity raise blood sugar, blunt metabolism, and can even shorten your lifespan. And, sorry, one workout a day doesn't undo the damage. The fix is simple: break up sitting with movement. Stand up at least once an hour, walk for ten minutes after meals, or do a few squats or stretches between calls or each time you go to the bathroom. Small, consistent bouts of movements can make a bigger impact than you think.

...eating vegan or plant-based?

Plant-based has a great ring to it, but the label doesn't automatically mean healthy. Oreos, French fries, and many fake meats are technically plant-based and technically vegan, too. Nutrition based on real plants (fruits, veggies, beans, nuts, seeds) is consistently linked to better health outcomes. You don't need to go 100 percent vegan to benefit. Shifting toward more actual plants helps; leaning on processed meat substitutes can backfire. Focus on real, whole foods, not the marketing language.

...the Carnivore Diet?

The Carnivore Diet is exactly what it sounds like—only animal products, no plants. Advocates say it's cleaner and point to plant anti-nutrients (like lectins and oxalates) as proof that vegetables are harmful. The reality? There are zero long-term studies on this diet, and cutting out entire food groups creates nutrient gaps, especially fiber and water-soluble vitamins. Yes, some plant compounds can irritate digestion in sensitive people, and most are neutralized by cooking. Carnivore might help some people short-term, but it's incredibly restrictive, rarely sustainable, and requires a greater commitment to getting the full range of nutrients the body needs.

...taking the easy way out?

Making healthy habits harder than they need to be is a recipe for burnout. The real easy way out isn't a magic pill; it's setting up your environment to make healthful choices simple and automatic (think: setting out workout clothes, pre-chopping veggies, or using reminders). No one wins for making it harder. Build systems that make the healthy thing the easiest thing to do.

...creatine?

Creatine isn't a steroid; it's a compound your body makes from amino acids and stores in muscle, heart, and brain cells for quick energy. Supplementing (three to five grams/day of creatine monohydrate) can improve muscle strength, speed recovery, support cognitive health, and even lower blood lipids. It's especially helpful if you do high-intensity exercise, want to maintain muscle as you age, or are at risk of sarcopenia. Creatine draws water into muscles (not fat), so don't confuse a slight increase on the scale with "getting bulky." Stick to recommended doses—more isn't better—and talk to your doctor if you have kidney or liver concerns.

...red light therapy?

Red light therapy (also called photobiomodulation) uses low-wavelength red or near-infrared light to stimulate cellular energy and may boost healing, collagen production, circulation, and reduce inflammation. Research suggests it can help with wound healing, some skin concerns, and even mood, but studies are still small and early. If you try it, follow the device instructions, aim for ten to twenty minutes per session a few times per week, and treat it as a complement to, not a replacement for, foundational health habits. (P.S. From what I've seen, the benefits only last as long as you keep doing it.)

...rice cakes?

Rice cakes are essentially empty carbs: little protein, fiber, or quality fat, so they don't keep you full and can spike blood sugar if eaten alone. If you love them, choose the plain versions with minimal ingredients, then top with protein and healthy fat (like nut butter or avocado) to balance the carbs. Or crumble a couple over soup or salad for crunch instead of making them the main event.

...food guilt?

Guilt is the extra seasoning we sprinkle on when we make choices out of alignment with our goals. Intentional choices (even indulgent ones) don't carry guilt; it's the mindless ones that do. Next time you feel it might creep in after eating/drinking something, pause and ask, *Why am I choosing this? How will I feel after? Am I okay with that?* If the answer is yes, enjoy it and move on. Journaling those moments can also help you spot patterns and adjust without shame.

...muscle weighing more than fat?

A pound is a pound, whether it's muscle or fat. The difference is density: a pound of muscle takes up less space than a pound of fat, so your body can look smaller and more toned even if the scale doesn't budge. Focus on body composition (measurements, body fat percent, and how you feel) instead of just the number on the scale.

...food porn?

Food porn is anything—cooking shows, commercials, Instagram feeds—that triggers cravings you didn't have a minute ago. It's not about shame; it's about awareness. Notice what sets you off and make a plan: watch Food Network only at the gym (I did this in college), swap cooking shows for competitions (they were less triggering for me), or unfollow accounts that make you want to dive into the pantry. Self-awareness turns mindless cravings into mindful choices.

...hunger?

Hunger isn't a moral failing; it's just your body's way of saying it needs energy or nutrients. True (homeostatic) hunger builds gradually and makes a variety of foods sound appealing. Learn your early signs, such as irritability, brain fog, trouble concentrating, or a dip in energy, so you can eat before you're hangry. Focus on nutrient-dense meals with protein and fiber to stay satisfied.

...cravings?

Also, not a moral failing. Cravings are different from hunger. They're a strong desire for a particular food, often driven by your brain's reward system rather than actual energy needs. They can be triggered by stress, boredom, or eating lots of ultra-processed, sweet, or salty foods. Sometimes cravings come from a lack of nutrients and the body signaling to get its needs met (sugar cravings are often associated with insufficient protein). Instead of white-knuckling it, pause and ask if another option would truly satisfy, or enjoy a small amount of what you're craving and move on.

...cheat days or cheat meals?

The word "cheat" sets you up for guilt and extremes. It turns one indulgent choice into either a full-day binge or a week of "making up" for it. And spoiler: cheat days and meals are not the definition or example of balance. They are, in fact, just as much on/off, good/bad, black/white as every diet. Instead, aim to keep the pendulum in the gray area: Make intentional choices, enjoy them, and keep going with your healthful habits. Food isn't good or bad, it's fuel and joy. When you remove the idea of cheating, you stop the punishment/reward cycle and create true harmony.

...alkaline water?

Alkaline water is trendy. Your body already works hard to keep its pH balanced. Drinking it might temporarily change the pH of your mouth or urine, but it won't alkalize your blood. If you enjoy it, stick to naturally alkaline spring water and use it as an occasional option; don't make it your only source of hydration. For me, there's no need to pay more for this water.

...plant milk?

Plant milks often have less protein than dairy, and many are sweetened or heavily processed. Read labels and choose the one that fits your needs. Unsweetened almond or oat milk might work as a creamer. If you want protein, stick to dairy or soy.

...cooling rice after cooking it?

Yes, cooking and cooling rice, potatoes, and even some pastas increases their resistant starch content. Resistant starch acts like fiber, feeding healthy gut bacteria, improving blood sugar control, and helping you feel fuller longer. After cooking, chill them for at least 12 to 24 hours, then eat cold or reheat; the benefits of resistant starch remain.

...olive oil?

Olive oil is a monounsaturated fat packed with polyphenols—antioxidants that help reduce inflammation, protect heart health, and support immunity. Not all olive oils are equal. Extra virgin (EVOO) has the highest polyphenol content, while light, pure, or refined olive oils have little to none. Always read labels; many bottles are blends with cheaper oils. Use EVOO raw (for salad dressings and drizzling) or for light sautéing. Its smoke point is ~325°F, so for roasting or high-heat cooking, use avocado oil instead.

...oatmeal?

Oatmeal can be a great source of fiber, but the less processed, the better. Instant and quick-cooking oats are more likely to spike blood sugar, while old-fashioned or steel-cut oats are digested more slowly and keep you fuller longer. Be sure to pair oats with protein, fiber, and quality fat (like nuts) for a balanced meal, and skip tossing them in a smoothie where they essentially become flour.

...air fryers?

Air fryers are a healthier alternative to deep frying because they use hot air and only a little oil, which cuts back on unhealthy trans and saturated fats. But they're not magic. Cooking proteins at high dry heat (like in an air fryer) can increase advanced glycation end products (AGEs), compounds linked to inflammation and aging. Use your air fryer for the occasional homemade sweet potato fries or veggie crisping, but be careful letting it become a daily habit for all your meals. It's a tool for moderation, not a license to eat fried foods every day.

...reading labels?

Food labels can be confusing and sometimes misleading. Focus on what the food gives you, not just what to avoid, which means understanding the quality of calories vs the total number. Look for protein (7 grams ≈ 1 ounce), at least 5 grams of fiber, and single-digit net carbs (total carbs − fiber − sugar alcohols - glycerin). Watch for hidden trans fats (look for "hydrogenated," "hydrolyzed," "modified," or "fractionated" in the ingredients), and take note of the serving sizes. Short ingredient lists you can pronounce usually win, and marketing claims like "gluten-free," "light," or "whole grain" don't necessarily mean the product is healthy.

...wearable tech (Fitbit, Apple Watch, Oura Ring, etc.)?

Wearables are great tools for spotting patterns, and they're not perfect. They may motivate you to move and give a relative sense of progress, yet metrics like calories burned, body fat percentage, and even sleep stages are often estimates. Use them for trends and relative assessments, not absolutes. Are you more active this week than last, sleeping better, recovering faster? If something consistently looks off (like heart rate or sleep quality), bring the data to your doctor or coach for context and action steps. Above all, be careful that the device doesn't replace listening to your body.

...collagen?

Collagen is the most abundant protein in the human body. It supports skin, joints, and bone health, but it's not a complete protein. If you're using it for protein, make sure you're also getting other sources like chicken, fish, or legumes. Look for Type I and Type III hydrolyzed collagen for skin, joint, and bone health benefits, plus better absorption.

...Ozempic and other GLP-1 medications?

These drugs (like Ozempic, Wegovy, and Mounjaro) were designed for type 2 diabetes but are now widely used for weight loss. They suppress appetite and slow digestion, but the weight lost often includes significant muscle mass, and long-term effects remain unknown. If you're considering them, work closely with a doctor and also with a coach, because decreasing the number on the scale doesn't necessarily equate to improved, long-term health and doesn't resolve underlying causes. Prioritize strength training, protein, and vitamin/mineral intake. Please know they're not a substitute for building sustainable habits.

...blue light?

We need blue light in the morning and during the day to set our circadian rhythm, support focus, and balance mood. Blocking it too early (with blue light–blocking glasses or heavy filters) can make you tired and disrupt your sleep-wake cycle. Save the blue light glasses and screen filters for evenings to help your body wind down for restful sleep.

...menopause/perimenopause?

This topic deserves more than a quick answer, but here's the short version: it's not in your head. The changes that come with this phase of life are real, and they rewrite a lot of what we thought we knew about our bodies. Yes, weight management gets trickier because estrogen is like your wiggle room, and in our 20s, we have more of both than we do in our 40s and beyond. Not only does it affect how much weight we carry, but also where we carry it. Your body also stops responding to workouts the way it used to. And weight? That's just one symptom out of hundreds. Another short answer: you're not doomed. This phase just calls for a deeper commitment and a more evolved toolkit than what worked for you in your 20s or 30s.

...weight loss resistance?

You're eating clean(ish), moving your body, hydrating, sleeping, and maybe even meditating. And the scale's not budging. It feels like your body's ignoring your effort. Weight loss resistance is often your body's way of protecting itself in response to chronic stress, low-quality sleep, inflammation, or metabolic shifts like insulin resistance. And what feels like "enough" sleep or "manageable" stress to you may not register the same way to your body. Alcohol can also quietly contribute. You don't have to cut it out completely, but it's worth checking in: is it helping or holding you back? If your progress has stalled, don't double down on what you've been doing; shift gears and support your body differently.

Conclusion
Okay, So It's a Little Complicated

Take a moment.

Seriously.

Right now.

Breathe in.

Let it go.

You just made it through a book that asked you to think differently about your body, your habits, your health, and probably yourself. That's not nothing. That's huge.

You've questioned rules you've followed for years. You've paused shame where it used to run the show. You've traded urgency for understanding. You've started to recognize when the wellness world is selling you nonsense and when your own body is telling you something real.

While this book is called *Uncomplicating Wellness*, we both know wellness isn't always simple. Or neat. Or linear. Yes, I've helped you clear the noise, ditch the shame, question the dogma, and stop chasing every shiny headline. And I know that doesn't mean everything gets easy.

Because now you're dealing with the real stuff. Your stuff.

Your body.

Your lifestyle.

Your goals, your hormones, your schedule, your family, your history, your stress, your sleep, your phase of life—and probably someone else's leftovers in your fridge.

This is where it gets nuanced. What works for one person doesn't necessarily work for another. What worked for you last year might not serve you next month. Your toolkit needs to shift because your context (a.k.a. your body, your lifestyle, and your priorities) keeps shifting.

And this is the part most wellness content skips. It's not complicated because you're doing it wrong. It's complicated because you're a living, breathing human being. And no static plan can keep up with a dynamic body and life.

So while this book gave you the lens, the clarity, the foundation, what comes next is more personal. It's the application. The adjustment. The part where you build a practice that fits your real life, not someone else's template.

From Knowing to Doing

This book offered you tools to see differently. And seeing clearly is only the beginning. Now comes the part where you experiment with things (maybe you already have, you overachiever, you). The part where you notice what works in your body—not just in theory, but in practice. Where you experiment, adjust, and maybe even mess it up a little (that's part of it, by the way).

Because knowing something isn't the same as living it. And living it looks different depending on the week, the season, the phase of life you're in, or the sleep you didn't get.

If you're thinking, *Okay, but now what?*—you're right where you want to be. Start with the area whose chapter had the most alarm bells going off in your mind. You know where to start. Play with one or two tweaks at a time. Track it, assess it, and adjust based on what you notice for you (the time when n=1 is the most powerful).

This is where application matters. This is where support helps. Maybe you want someone to walk through this with you. Maybe you want accountability. Maybe you want a place to ask the real questions and get answers that don't feel like another can of worms. That's what I do.

Whether it's one-on-one coaching, joining my group, or being part of a community where you can get your questions answered without judgment. This work gets easier when you don't do it alone. If you're ready to take what you've read and make it real in your own life, that's the next step. And I'd be honored to walk it with you.

What Comes Next (If You Want More)

You don't need to do this alone. You can. You've got the tools, the filter, the foundation. And if you're ready for the next layer? That's where I come in. There's a reason I coach, not because I think people need fixing, but because wellness in real life takes support. It takes troubleshooting. It takes someone to remind you what matters when life gets loud again. And honestly? It's just more doable (and more fun) when you've got someone in your corner.

If you're craving a personalized approach—something that meets your life, your hormones, your schedule—I work with clients 1:1. If you want community, accountability, and coaching that cuts through the fluff, my group programs and the Happy Healthy Hub membership are built precisely for that. And if you're more of the "give me the next book" type? I hear you. It's coming.

However, you want to keep going—there's a place for you. Check out www.asaladwithasideoffries.com/book for additional resources, to stay in touch, and more.

Plus, the *Salad with a Side of Fries* podcast brings you wellness without the weirdness every week for six years and counting...

You get to decide what's next. And when you're ready, I'll be here.

Acknowledgments

I'd like to thank French fries and cookie dough—two foods I'll never give up. Just kidding. Kinda. For real, though, now I get how people feel when they walk up to the podium to accept an award and are so afraid they'll leave someone out. More than that, I also know if you're reading this far, you likely know me, may recognize some names, and still, a list of people's names isn't interesting to anyone.

I'd be remiss if I didn't let you all know that I am who I am because of my family and friends. When I started my health coaching practice as a side hustle back in 2007, this book was not even a figment of my imagination. For every bit of excitement all you have shown along the way, I am eternally grateful. Not only are you all my biggest cheerleaders, you are my sounding board, my clients, my occasional podcast co-hosts, and everything in between.

I often describe myself as an insatiable student. To try to name every teacher, mentor, and colleague I've learned from is an impossible task. Many of you know who you are (yes, you), and many I may never meet. I am a sponge for all you share. We are all more and better because we continue to learn, question, and grow.

Let's all acknowledge the human body. The more I learn, the more I am in awe. It is an absolute miracle. And for as much as we know, as much as we understand it, I believe there is still so much yet to be discovered.

For this book specifically, the teams at Twin Flames Studios, Produce Your Podcast, and my team at Salad with a Side of

Fries —you all made this process light, fun, and, frankly, possible within the timeframe we did it. Sure, it was a lifetime in the making, and then a few months of consistent, focused effort.

Last but not least, you, dear reader, friend. You made it this far. Wow! I am humbled and honored. I can't wait to see all you do with everything shared here. Any progress you've already experienced, know that YOU did that, and you can continue. Your health is yours to create. What an absolute gift!

About the Author

Jenn Trepeck is a force of nature in the wellness space. She is an Optimal Health Coach, entrepreneur, and host of the award-winning podcast *Salad with a Side of Fries*. Known for her sharp insights, science-savvy coaching, and real-talk approach to nutrition and weight management, Jenn's passion for health stems from her saga of kicking her food issues and navigating the frustration of conflicting advice, fad diets, and diet culture.

Since becoming a coach in 2007, she has helped clients achieve lasting results by cutting through wellness overwhelm and focusing on what truly works. Her work has been recognized by *Podcast Magazine's* "40 Under 40," the International Women's Podcast Awards, and the Women Who Podcast Awards, and she is the winner of Ear Worthy's 2024 and 2025 Best Health Podcast and Best Independent Podcast.

With her signature blend of wit, science, and sanity, Jenn empowers people to trust their bodies, release perfectionism, and make health a sustainable, joyful part of real life.

When she's not coaching or recording, Jenn's usually at a Physique57 or A-List workout class, discovering NYC's hidden gem restaurants, or spending time with the people she loves.

www.ingramcontent.com/pod-product-compliance
Lightning Source LLC
Chambersburg PA
CBHW031433270326
41930CB00007B/683